MAXIMUM BRAINPOWER

MAXIMUM
BRAINPOWER

CHALLENGING THE BRAIN
FOR HEALTH AND WISDOM

Shlomo Breznitz

AND

Collins Hemingway

BALLANTINE BOOKS | NEW YORK

Published in the United States by Ballantine Books,
an imprint of The Random House Publishing Group,
a division of Random House, Inc., New York.

BALLANTINE and colophon are registered
trademarks of Random House, Inc.

ISBN 978-0-345-52614-4
eBook ISBN 978-0-345-52616-8

Printed in the United States of America on acid-free paper

www.ballantinebooks.com

246897531

FIRST EDITION

Book design by Casey Hampton

To Danny, Ruthie, and Nurit

Contents

Introduction

What does it say about the brain that three of the first five American presidents died on the Fourth of July?

What do schizophrenia, poetry, and corny jokes tell us about how we all learn?

What discussion about the nature of thought might logically tie together topics as diverse as financial trading, Middle East politics, and avian intelligence operatives?

How can we know something and not know it at the same time?

Welcome to the wonderful world of the brain.

And welcome to *Maximum Brainpower: Challenging the Brain for Health and Wisdom,* a book that seeks to answer all of these questions, and many more besides. Brainpower is our ability to gather the many aspects of our intelligence and apply them in practical ways. By maximizing our brainpower, we can keep our brains sharp and cognitively fit, especially—but not only—as we age. This is not about doing better on brain teasers or brain exercises. Nor is it about being able to do crossword puzzles in ink instead of pencil or solving logic problems or puzzles. It's about becoming more capable in our daily lives: being able to accurately assess and navigate the world, knowing what to pay attention to and what not to, thinking and planning ahead, and making the right decisions. It is about changing *the inherent way we perceive and respond to the world.*

Most of us recognize that a fit brain is probably the most important contributor to a long, healthy, and active life. And, as a result, most of us fear Alzheimer's disease, stroke, and other ailments that might break down or damage our brains. Many adults have borne witness to the failing mental health of their parents, and Baby Boomers are beginning to stumble through their own "senior moments." Yet relatively little in-depth, scientifically accurate, and easy-to-understand information on cognitive fitness is available to the general reader. This book intends to provide it.

Because our minds are the core of our existence, understanding the brain may be the most important and fundamental task before us. I have spent my professional career as a psychologist and professor studying many aspects of thought and behavior. And for a decade I have researched cognitive fitness; work that culminated in my founding of CogniFit, a company devoted to improving cognitive vitality in a substantive way. After many years, the concept of improving and protecting our mental capabilities has begun to enter into the mainstream—though sometimes it has been explained or promoted superficially. *Maximum Brainpower* brings to the thoughtful person the most up-to-date knowledge of the brain and its functions. It shows us how we can all achieve the cognitive vitality to improve our personal and professional lives.

Filled with pragmatic examples and scenarios, *Maximum Brainpower* addresses the major issues that we face in our daily lives: problems of personal growth, family relationships, and important social and cultural matters. This book also exposes the inherent dangers of a brain that at times is too quick to change its mind and at other times cannot seem to change at all.

Maximum Brainpower is divided into five major sections.

Part I: Maximum Brainpower in the Real World uses many examples from the real world to show how cognitive fitness is important in unexpected, subtle, and critical ways. We focus on the role that experience plays in learning, and how it can set us up for cognitive failure. The very mental abilities that provide our creativity can also lead to rigidity of thought and cognitive stagnation.

Part II: The Case for Heavy Mental Lifting demonstrates the importance of challenging our brains. Doing so helps us develop and maintain cognitive fitness, with benefits accruing biologically and psychologically. Included are strategies for building cognitive reserves at any age and how these reserves can benefit us.

Part III: Change as a Pathogen addresses the basic quandary of mental fitness. We need change to stimulate the brain; but change causes stress, which brings its own kinds of harm. Stress can damage our mental and physical health, but a lack of stress will lead us into cognitive rigidity and decline. These chapters describe the complex interactions of stress on our psyches and our bodies and methods for reducing the negative impact.

Part IV: What to Do explores the ways in which we can develop our cognitive reserves without being overwhelmed by stress. Spanning our careers, education, and personal lives, the chapters in this section show the need for new approaches to get us outside the comfort zone of routine life: new ways to view the world, new approaches to thinking, and a consistent regimen to build the brain.

Part V: Thinking Ahead envisions the way the world will look if we all fully develop cognitive fitness. The chapters in this section also examine how we can ensure that cognitively fit people develop the personal and social connections necessary to stay grounded in an increasingly chaotic society.

Maximum Brainpower is for anyone who is genuinely curious about the world in which we live, who enjoys introspection, and who longs for a greater understanding of their own interior world. And cognitive health is important to all audiences of any age. Young people can improve their studying skills, driving skills, and their ability to handle risky situations. The elderly can recover mental capacity. People who have survived physical brain trauma can substantively recover their mental and physical abilities. Businesses can improve their employees' performance by developing an understanding of how the brain learns and adapts—and how business routines literally map the mind into uncreative patterns.

Who we are, after all, *is* a manifestation of our brain activity. We *are* our cognitive life: our perceptions, our thoughts and memories, our personalities. *Maximum Brainpower* undertakes an exploration of the private mental world that is, in poetic terms, the seat of our hearts and souls. This book explores the place where our *humanness* and our *humanity* both reside.

PART I

MAXIMUM BRAINPOWER IN THE REAL WORLD

WHY BRAINPOWER IS NOT ABOUT HOW WE DO ON TESTS BUT HOW WE DO IN LIFE

ONE

Why Experts Know Nothing

John Smith is a tall, lanky Londoner with a flair for silk ties. He works in an office amid piles of coffee cups and soft-drink cans—anything with caffeine. He stares all day long at a wall of computer screens. John makes millions of dollars a day, and he has no idea how.

John's story is the story of the expert—the person who has so much ability and experience that he or she finds quick solutions to complicated problems that vex the rest of us. We all know experts. The auto mechanic who in ten minutes fixes an engine that stumps everyone else in the garage. The cook who with a single sip identifies the one missing ingredient that will make a good soup great. The engineer who draws by hand an airfoil design as efficient as that produced by a computer. The doctor who plucks the correct diagnosis out of thin air, unsupported by tests and scans (think television's Dr. House, only with nicer bedside manners).

Experts process a problem through the vast amounts of knowledge and experience they have accumulated, and out pops an answer—usually the correct one, sometimes an unexpected one. I met John, a currency trader, before the introduction of the euro, at a time when every European country still had its own currency. Most large companies hold and trade different currencies in order to pay bills in local currencies and to avoid being caught with excessive holdings in case one currency's value declines. Financial institutions actively trade in currency as they would in any stock or commodity, in the hopes of making money by determining whether a particular currency will go up or down.

John was one of those institutional mavericks who was exceedingly good at what he did. His specialty was buying and selling U.S. dollars against the German mark. Known as "the money factory," he brought in millions of dollars in profits every month. The large international financial institution where he worked feared that competitors would steal him away, or that he'd simply retire. He had made so much money for himself and for the company over the years that he no longer needed to work.

How did this trader do it? How did he regularly bet on the right currency? The company leaders decided that perhaps a smart psychologist might be able to tell them, which is where I came in. By gaining insights into John's intellectual methods and analytical processes, they hoped to protect themselves against his possible departure and to learn how they might train others to achieve similar results.

For days I sat next to John on the trading floor amid his computers and clutter. There were other traders in the middle of the floor, calling out offers to buy or sell. It was very, very busy, and very, very dull. Hour after hour, we watched the screens as the dollar and mark went up and down against each other. I saw every uptick and downtick that he did. I heard the same announcements. We watched news on economic and political activity all over the world on the "tickers" streaming by on the screens. Over the course of several days, he made modest trades, but nothing spectacular. Very boring stuff. A currency trader *must* be well paid to sit through this kind of tedium all of his life.

Then, one day, he was suddenly electrified. He held up his hand, flashing his fingers to signal "five," then "three." I scanned the screens. I zoned in on every word the sellers on the floor were saying. Nothing obvious had happened, and yet—within a few seconds—John had bought eight million marks! Before long, the

value of the mark began to rise. By the close of trading, this gentleman and his company had made a very tidy profit.

By then, John and I had become friendly. Over a few pints of
Guinness after work, I asked him why he had bought marks at that
particular moment. I expected a technical analysis relating to economic news or monetary policy. Or perhaps, like an experienced
chess player who has seen about every gambit imaginable, John had
detected a series of clever moves by other traders and was able to
exploit them for his own gain. His answer?

"I suddenly felt," he said, "*The mark wants to go up.*"

Say again?

"It was a feeling. 'It feels like the mark wants to go up.' "

We talked for quite a while. I don't believe he was putting me on,
or putting me off. He genuinely could not explain his instinct to buy
marks at that particular moment. It was a feeling. He could not say
how or where he could "feel" it. He just could. He was influenced
by something he couldn't verbalize. Perhaps tension crept into the
voices of the brokers on the trading floor. Perhaps there was some
pattern in the movements of rates that he picked up unconsciously.
Perhaps, at some unconscious level, he recalled a similar pattern
from a few weeks or months before. Perhaps his own large pur-
chase, coming out of nowhere, created a mini-stampede that drove
the price of the mark higher. But people bought and sold marks all
day, often in large volumes. How did he know when the time was
right to make his move? He didn't know. The effort to understand
his process was a total waste of time.

My shadowing project ended a short time later when the bank
was sold, but I do not believe I would have learned anything more
if I had remained by John's side for a year, or even ten. I would have
experienced a great deal of boredom for nothing. He was right
about when to trade currency. That is all there was to say.

John's inability to explain his strategy is no isolated example.
Gerd Gigerenzer, in his book *Gut Feelings*, writes about police officers who can instantly spot a drug carrier in a crowd on the basis
of nothing more than a "hunch." Malcolm Gladwell, in his book
Blink, describes art experts who can, at a glance, tell whether a

statue is an authentic work or a forgery. They cannot explain how they know. Gigerenzer speaks of a gut feeling—an unconscious, immediate "fast and frugal" aspect of cognition that is strong enough to act upon even though we are not fully aware of why. Gladwell calls this ability "thin slicing," describing it as an automated, accelerated ability to find patterns in a small amount of information. Experts are able to reduce a complex situation to a simple one very fast through some process of unconscious inference.

This chapter explores the cognitive processes of experts such as John to figure out how their expertise emerges. It is the beginning of our story about how the brain works, how it is shaped by experience, and how experience can be good or bad depending on our response.

OF SOLDIERS AND ROADSIDE BOMBS

People who work in harm's way learn to rely on the indefinable instincts that mark the expert, the "feelings" that do not come from the conscious verbal pathways that we commonly identify with "thinking." These instincts probably stem from the more primitive pathways of the brain, the parts of the limbic system—the "old brain"—that kept our ancient forebears alive when there was no time to evaluate situations in a calm and reflective manner. Police officers and soldiers in particular learn to "trust their gut" on dangerous streets and roadways.

In Iraq and Afghanistan, improvised explosive devices (IEDs, or roadside bombs) have caused more than half of all of the deaths of American and coalition soldiers plus untold numbers of civilians. Several hundred other IED attacks occur *every month* elsewhere in the world. The United States alone has been spending more than two billion dollars a year trying to counter IEDs, using heavier armor, spy aircraft, ground robots, and a variety of electronic devices to discover and disable them. Yet there have only been two consistently reliable approaches to finding roadside bombs, neither of which is sophisticated. The first is getting information from locals about where the IEDs are planted. The second is relying on soldiers who spot the devices from moving vehicles.

It turns out that a small number of combat veterans have an uncanny knack for detecting these bombs. Some of the signs of an IED require nothing more than close observation. A normally busy street is deserted. A pile of debris appears along a road that was recently cleared. Vehicles are left in unusual places for no apparent reason. At times, however, a "bomb-sniffing" soldier simply has a "feeling"—like our currency trader—that something has changed. Once a bomb is discovered it is possible to speculate on what small clue the observer might have spotted, but at the crucial moment, it is usually only a single soldier—often the same one—who is able to detect something that's amiss. Why?

One clue may come from experiments involving pigeons.

OF PIGEONS, PAINTINGS, AND PHOTOS

Birds as a whole, and pigeons in particular, have great perceptual skills. Pigeons can distinguish differences in geometric shapes, colors, and patterns, and between classes of items such as cats, chairs, cars, and flowers. They can recognize themselves in mirrors, as only a few other species can. In one study, pigeons learned to discriminate between paintings by Picasso and Monet. After training, the birds were able to identify the painters' work, correctly categorizing paintings that they had never seen before. Eventually, they even learned to pick out paintings that were either cubist (Picasso's style) or impressionist (Monet's). Their success was identical to that of college students who were given the same amount of instruction. Not bad for bird brains.

Humans have recognized the military value of these birds for some time. First employed as battlefield messengers, pigeons were used for aerial surveillance in World War I. (These efforts proved problematic because the heavy cameras strapped to the birds often forced them to walk home.) Aided by an extra set of color-sensing cones in their retinas (which mammals lack), pigeons have keen eyesight, and it was this ability that first turned them into intelligence operatives.

Even in an age of high-tech wizardry and high-resolution imaging, one of the most difficult intelligence challenges is identifying military equipment or personnel in photographs. Targets of interest are often hidden. Among dozens or hundreds of photographs covering many square miles of territory, where does an analyst begin to look? Knowing that pigeons had been trained to distinguish "tree" from "not tree," some intelligence agents decided to go one step further and determine whether pigeons could differentiate between "natural" and "manmade."

The birds were shown two sets of photographs, one containing one class of objects, and the other containing a different class of objects. There were all natural objects in one set of photos and manmade objects interspersed with natural objects in the other set. Simply put: natural versus manmade. If the photo was natural and the birds pecked on the left lever, they received a reward of food. If the photo included manmade objects and the birds pecked on the right lever, they received a reward of food. Any other choice left them without a treat.

Before long, the pigeons were able to correctly identify "natural" versus "manmade." They continued to be able to distinguish the difference, even as the manmade objects became less and less obvious. Eventually, with their keen eyesight, the pigeons were able to detect manmade objects that were as inconspicuous in the photographs they were shown as deliberately hidden military hardware would be in a desert or forest. The point, though, is not that these birds have impressive eyesight. It's that they can learn to generalize— to identify new examples within one class or to distinguish members of different classes. The pigeon brain is twenty grams in size, *one-seventieth* the size of a human brain. Yet lo and behold this tiny little brain can learn a very subtle rule, *even though that rule is never explicitly defined*! What is the definition of "manmade" that a bird can understand? Are manmade patterns, even irregular ones, far more symmetrical to a pigeon brain than natural patterns? Can it discern differences in texture or reflectivity? We do not know. We know only that brains far less sophisticated than ours can see, conceptualize, and react to things that are virtually imperceptible.

The pigeon's impressive perception lies below the level of verbalizing thought. It may be that humans have similar abilities buried deep within the brain. This would explain why some soldiers can see things in their mind's eye that others cannot. Like pigeons, certain people may be able to recognize "danger" among all the clutter of a ramshackle street or a rural setting. Soldiers who are the best at spotting IEDs usually grew up in either perilous urban neighborhoods or in rural areas where they hunted. In other words, they were raised in environments in which they needed to be constantly vigilant. One soldier, a deer hunter from Michigan, detected a three-inch clothes pin at thirty yards and recognized it as a bomb trigger.

The question this raises, oddly enough, is whether the military should try to teach bomb-finding skills to soldiers who lack this natural ability. Like most other experts, the soldiers who are good at finding bombs may not be able to articulate why. More important, the other soldiers could potentially be better off learning to develop their own "sixth sense" than to learn four or five particular things to look for. *The very lack of training may open the mind to new stimuli.* By engaging their conscious minds with a memorized list of possible signs of IEDs, the soldiers could be disengaging their unconscious minds, reducing the level of visual and mental alertness that might best serve them.

This point is supported by an experiment devised by Donald Spence. Subjects were told that the study was nothing more than a test of memory. In reality, it was a test of the brain's ability to make unconscious connections. Subjects were presented with a list of words and asked to recount the ones they remembered. Spence arranged the words in such a way that about half of them had a common but undeclared denominator. The common denominator was the word "cheese," which was itself on the list along with other associated words—"ripe," "smell," "blue," and so on. The list also contained words not normally associated with cheese.

Spence found an intriguing dichotomy. If the subject recalled the actual word "cheese," he or she recalled fewer related words. And he or she recalled fewer related words *after* identifying the word "cheese" than before. But if the subject did *not* recall the word "cheese," he or she remembered *more* cheese-related words. The result seems counterintuitive. Wouldn't we recall more related words after hitting upon the central idea? No—because after finding the solution, the brain stops searching.

Like the pigeons, these humans were able to sense that, within the seemingly random list of words, there was an undefined central concept ("cheesiness"). Once a subject identified the central idea consciously, the problem was closed, the brain stopped searching for connections, and fewer related concepts registered. But if a subject could not detect the central idea—could not "solve" the problem—the brain kept working and more things connected to cheese surfaced in awareness. The less that surfaced consciously, the more the brain kept plugging away. This led to the recall of many more related words. On the topic of the restricting effect of awareness, Spence's study sparked a series of research that all supported the same basic point: Sometimes we are better off not knowing the rule, because then we are more open to all related possibilities. These studies indicate that mental processes of which we are not even aware are in some ways much deeper and more interesting than the ones of which we are aware.

OF BRAINS, COMPUTERS, AND LEARNING

Enormous effort is being poured into the development of pattern recognition software by all kinds of organizations for all kinds of needs. In addition to the problem of detecting hidden military equipment, law enforcement agencies want facial recognition software to help them pick criminals and terrorists out of a crowd. Businesses want to understand facial expressions to gauge consumer reactions to sales promotions. High-tech companies want to develop computers that react to both gestures and expressions. Despite impressive advancements in gesture recognition, progress in this field has overall been slow. Some computer systems can recognize users' faces well enough to be used at security checkpoints, but their effectiveness is limited. They compare a person's face to either a small database of users or an image in the microchip of the person's passport or security card.

Larger scale systems, in which a computer is tasked with picking a specific face out of thousands of faces that are at different angles and in different lighting conditions, have generally failed. Yet humans can recognize one person among thousands at a football stadium, sometimes with only a brief or partial glance. The reason is that the brain and the computer function in fundamentally different ways. The brain can fill in missing information and use partial cues to recognize a face or solve a problem. Computer programs, on the other hand, require a high degree of precision in how they are programmed. The computer must know exactly what it is looking for, and that problem brings in a huge number of variables. How can a human being tell a computer to fill in certain kinds of data when he or she does not know what kind of data to insert, or how? The brain does this for us, without conscious thought. All of us are experts at pattern recognition. We are particularly adept at finding a complete pattern despite missing data. This skill can be seen in something as simple as the phrase "C n Y u Und rst nd Th se W rds?" or in the abbreviated phraseology of texting. We suffer from the limitations of the expert, though: We lack the ability to explain how we achieve our ends.

Inherent differences between the computer and the brain involve not just perception but calculation. Computers are rule based. The rules must be precise or the computer spits out nonsense, as every beginning programmer quickly learns. Since Descartes, many philosophers have assumed that human thought follows the same kind of rule-based logic. In the Age of Reason, the brain was viewed as little more than an information processing system. And it's true that we are quite good at rule-based thinking. We follow a series of logical steps when we begin from a premise and, on the basis of rules, work logically up from the specific to the general; or when we begin with a general set of facts and, on the basis of rules, work logically down from the general to the specific. Our ability with this type of thought has led to the development of fields such as mathematics, geometry, physics, and, of course, computer science. Our languages are rule-based as well. We are born with a brain that appears compelled to construct language.

However, there is another way in which we acquire knowledge. Case learning, which may actually be the primary way in which we learn, is likely the key to why experts have trouble explaining what they do. This "illogical" manner of learning on a case-by-case basis instead of by rules has frustrated logicians for as long as they have written books. Socrates spoke to the experts in ancient Athens to try to understand the rules they used to master their fields. He asked the priest Euthyphro to explain how we can recognize piety. Rather than state any rules, Euthyphro gave examples from history and mythology as instances of pious acts. Socrates had the same problem elucidating answers from craftsmen, poets, and politicians. They could all give instances but not rules. He concluded sardonically that experts knew nothing, and neither did he. Plato followed with a gentler interpretation, that experts had learned their skills in a previous life, now forgotten.

Philosopher Hubert L. Dreyfus uses this anecdote as a launching point for the theme developed here, that experts use something other than logic to achieve their ends. Dreyfus says that people master a skill *initially* by following a set of rules and *later* by using knowledge acquired situationally, through a number of particular instances—through experience. By the time we become an expert— at chess, at driving a car—we no longer follow rules. We establish the goal we want to achieve ("win the match," "drive to New York"), and then canvass the instances stored in our head to determine the ideal strategy. Whereas the proficient performer makes conscious decisions, the expert pulls from among thousands of special cases in order to act quickly and intuitively.

Gigerenzer, in his book on hunches, shows the difference between the logical consciousness of the neophyte and the non-logical non-consciousness of the expert by citing studies of golfers. A poor golfer who takes more time to think about a shot will generally do better, but an expert golfer who takes more time will generally do worse. The reason is that the expert's unconscious already knows what to do (thanks to what golf instructors call "muscle memory"). Thinking too much interferes with an ability that is already developed.

Because we have already compared the brain to a computer, let us return to software programming for a clarifying example. A software engineer stuck with code that is too large or slow can prune unused logical constructs to wring small amounts of improvement here and there. (Such compression can be done automatically by computer programs in a process known as optimization.) To achieve dramatic performance gains, however, the software engineer must devise an entirely new approach, one that solves the problem in a totally different way. Such solutions, where twenty lines of code might replace two hundred, and performance improves geometrically, are considered "elegant." An intuitive leap to a new solution is far more likely to come from case learning than from the application of rules—unless the rule is "think of something else." We have no way to formulate a way, rule-based or otherwise, to tell a computer when to seek such a leap, or how to achieve it.

This brings us to two conclusions. First, we should not use experts to set up an expert system, especially computerized ones, because *experts have no idea how they do what they do.* Except for their specific answers (which are usually quite valuable), we do not learn any larger lessons that can help us tackle other questions. It's as though we've received the answers to a math test without understanding how they were derived. The correct person to set up an expert system is someone who is highly proficient but not quite expert, for that person can still articulate his or her principles and methodologies.

Second, expert systems are themselves problematic if the goal is to match human thinking and behavior. Web search engines, text-analysis systems, and software that recommends medical treatments are examples of useful expert systems. In general, these tools canvass far more information than people can, and much more rapidly. But when it comes to emulating actual thought, expert systems—in the form of artificial intelligence (AI)—remain in the infant stage. It has taken decades and hundreds of millions of dollars for a computer to occasionally beat a human world champion at chess, or the top human contestants at the game *Jeopardy!* In the latter case, IBM's Watson—with 2,800 processors, two hundred million pages of content, and six million rules—won at *Jeopardy!,* not because it got more answers right but primarily because its electronic reaction time was faster than the human reaction time. It usually hit the answer buzzer first.

Research has shown that challenges involving vision and language cannot be solved with "neat," scientifically provable, rule-based logic. New approaches to AI programming have been dubbed "scruffy," because they must be built not on logic but painfully, case by case. The now derogatory term "hacking" was originally used to define the software changes that AI programmers had to make in order to obtain intelligent behavior from software when logic broke down. With computers doubling in power every two years, they will have more connections than the human brain within two decades. Things will get interesting then. For now, though, AI systems cannot distinguish between an apple and a tomato. And by mentally mapping obstacles and pathways faster and more accurately, a four-year-old child can still outmaneuver the best-engineered robots in a race around the living room.

We will know that artificial intelligence has come of age when computers master the art of commonsense behavior in the real world. "Common sense" is the brain's unique ability to make sense of confusing patterns by filling in missing information, using partial cues and pulling together relevant data from a large set of individual cases. Whether the subjects are pigeons, soldiers, or ordinary people, our brains sometimes develop an organizing principle without us knowing what it is. This ability to find solutions buried in our experience is a hallmark of human creativity. And it is the expert's greatest strength.

As adults, everyone becomes an expert in life. We all regularly have unconscious, instantaneous inferences about people and situations. We simply know things without being able to account for that knowledge. Our ability to "know more than we can tell" has been examined in psychology for more than four decades. Richard Nisbett and Timothy Wilson discovered something even more curious: We also "tell more than we can know." That is, when we describe what we think, we often say things that are provably wrong and thus "more" than we could possibly know. What we think, and what we *think* we think, are often at odds. In several different clinical tests, subjects were given a stimulus to see whether it changed their behavior, whether they were aware of the change, and whether they could correctly identify the stimulus causing the change. As it turns out, they were pretty much clueless about all of these things. They often changed their behavior without being aware of it and without knowing the cause! For example, writing an essay on a topic opposite to their personal point of view often shifted subjects' attitudes toward the other side. Despite post-essay follow-ups showing a distinct shift, most people denied any change at all.

Test subjects were also usually unaware of the stimulus causing the change in their behavior. Insomniacs, for example, took longer to fall asleep when given a pill they thought would relax them, and fell asleep faster when given a pill they thought would stimulate them. Neither pill had any actual medical effect. After taking a "relaxation" pill that did nothing, subjects unconsciously credited their still-alert state to hyperactivity, making it harder for them to drift off. Having taken an "arousal" pill, subjects unconsciously ascribed their continued alertness to the pill, relaxed, and went to sleep faster.

Until they were told, none of the insomniac subjects realized that their sleep patterns had changed. Then they attributed the wrong reasons for it—bringing up everything except for the pills. None of them could believe that the pills, which were said to have one effect, would have had the opposite effect, all because of an unconscious rationalization process inside of their heads. These studies indicate that after we experience a change of mind or behavior we look back, analyze the change, and generate a plausible reason, which may or may not be correct.

Cognition is a much deeper and subtler process than we might suppose. The remarkably fast and inexplicable manner in which experts reach their conclusions can illuminate the untapped potential in all of us. Another lesson is that we may be at our most creative *when we do not understand what is going on*! Yet humanity's cognitive strengths can also be our biggest weaknesses. Our ability to find similarity in things, to find hidden patterns, and to "fill in the blanks" can lead us into mental traps. Experts do not, in fact, maximize brainpower. They do very much the opposite. They become brilliant in a narrow range of mental activity. (The joke is that experts are people who know more and more about less and less until eventually they know everything about nothing.) At the peak of their abilities, they lack mental challenge. Reliance on what they already know causes them to run the risk of rapid cognitive deterioration. The next chapters show how quickly the piercing insight of the expert can become trapped in the tomb of experience.

===== **LESSONS IN BRAINPOWER** =====

- Experts cannot explain what they do, because they do not make their decisions based on rule-based logic.
- Though much of human learning and knowledge is based on rules, the primary method by which humans learn is through the accumulation of experience.
- The difference between human thought and computer calculation is that humans can comprehend a situation by filling in the blanks when information is missing—as it usually is in the real world.
- Our conscious minds often have no idea what we are learning unconsciously.

TWO

The False Lessons of False Alarms

Surrounded by hostile neighbors, Israel is one of the most vigilant nations in the world. It has sophisticated and aggressive intelligence services to detect serious threats and an advanced air force and highly trained and well-equipped army to respond to them. In 1973, as the country was preparing for its holiest day—Yom Kippur—it believed it was too strong to be attacked. Yet when the Israelis awoke on the morning of October 6, they found that Egyptian troops had breached the country's southern border and Syrian troops were advancing from the north. Thus began a bloody three-week conflict in which Israel's very existence hung in the balance.

How could a country, embattled since its creation, not notice that its biggest military antagonists were preparing for a major war? The story of the Yom Kippur War is not a story of carelessness or ineptitude on the part of the Israelis. It is a story of the dangers of experience. Israel could not believe that war was imminent because of one of the most insidious forms of experience: false alarms. The Yom Kippur War is not so much a military history as a psychological history. It is an example of what happens when our amazing brains fill in the blanks with the wrong data and detect the wrong pattern in the mix of information.

Experience befuddled Israel because Egypt's President Anwar Sadat had threatened war numerous times since the Arab debacle in the Six-Day War of 1967, yet nothing had come of his saber rattling. In May and August of 1973, major Egyptian maneuvers caused Israel to mobilize its military, but no war came. Just before Yom Kippur, Egypt conducted exercises near the border again, then demobilized the troops that had been involved. All of these actions, along with an Egyptian misinformation campaign that indicated a lack of general military readiness, caused the Israeli intelligence service to discount other *significant* evidence of an imminent war. Even when King Hussein, fearful that Jordan would be drawn into the conflict, secretly flew to Tel Aviv to warn Prime Minister Golda Meir of the threat, the Israeli government did not act! The country failed to mobilize its troops until a few hours before the invasion. By then it was too late to repulse the initial attacks.

This one set of false experiences, now considered a classic example of military deception, was sufficient to fool an entire intelligence system and all of a country's senior decision makers. Yet the problem is not unique to one society or culture or to one moment in time. "The Boy Who Cried Wolf" is the famous cautionary tale of the little shepherd boy who falsely warns of a wolf so many times that the villagers ignore him when a real wolf comes along and feasts on him for dinner. The danger is so endemic that this fable exists in many forms around the world. In the real world, the problem is not that people create false alarms for their own amusement but that experience with a past false alarm distorts their view of reality.

People wonder why multiple government agencies and local residents failed to prepare for Hurricane Katrina in 2005. Why did the full-scale evacuation begin so late that more than 1,800 people died when the massive hurricane slammed into Louisiana and Mississippi? The reason is that the region has experienced a hurricane about once every three years for as long as anyone can remember. *Six* had hit the area in the decade leading up to Katrina. Almost every resident remembered these hurricanes, which had come and gone, once in a while causing damage, but never creating wholesale devastation. There was almost a perverse pride in ignoring the warnings . . . until it was too late.

My laboratory studies show that a *single* false alarm—in which "experience" teaches us to ignore danger signs—reduces the fear reaction to a subsequent similar threat significantly, by close to 50 percent. It is difficult to retain watchfulness when warnings prove wrong. Even after the brutal terrorist attacks of recent years— including 9/11 in the United States and later attacks in London, Madrid, Indonesia, and elsewhere—it is a demanding task to maintain vigilance against terrorist threats because of the number of false alarms that occur in between real ones. The biggest danger of the repeated warnings of potential flu pandemics is that we will be lulled into inaction—until *after* the disease has ravaged the world.

As individuals, we have trouble paying attention to personal matters—an unhappy boss, a child having problems in school, unsettling medical symptoms—if earlier, similar circumstances turned out okay. Many friends of mine had false alarms with one or two biopsies. They procrastinated on later checkups and eventually paid a heavy price. The problem with false alarms is inherent in the pattern recognition systems in our brain, which make it difficult for us to unlearn something, *especially if what needs to be unlearned gives us false comfort.*

CHANGING THE SHEPHERD'S SITUATION

Our traditional "cry wolf" story is about a boy who wanted to make fun of people by fooling them. In some forms of the story, the danger is not always a wolf. Sometimes it is another creature or another kind of threat. But structurally the story stays the same. Someone sets off a deliberate false alarm and eventually suffers dearly for it. The lesson—not to scream "danger!" unless we really mean it—has developed independently everywhere.

Variations of this story are even more frightening because they show just how diabolical this false alarm problem is. Consider the following scenario: One day the shepherd boy spots a wolf sneaking up on the village's sheep. The boy immediately shouts, "Come,

come, there is a wolf!" The villagers race to defend the flock, causing the wolf to flee before they can get there. To the shepherd, who
was frightened by the wolf, and to the wolf, who was frightened by
the villagers, it was no false alarm.

But from the villagers' point of view, the lack of a verifiable wolf
creates the perception of a false alarm. It does not matter that the
shepherd argues desperately that the wolf ran away before the villagers arrived. In terms of a loss of credibility, the next time the
shepherd cries wolf, only half the village will come. The very precautions that are taken against danger may be so effective that the
danger disappears and the incident registers as a false alarm.

There is a distinction here between two types of danger. The first
is naïve danger, which moves forward regardless of how the endangered responds. Naïve danger would include a natural disaster such
as a hurricane, flood, earthquake, or a plague or other biological
pestilence that has no personal motivation with regard to the target.
In fact, there is no target; there are merely those who happen to get
in the way. The second type of danger is adaptive danger, in which
defensive measures by the endangered party might reduce the
danger . . . or cause the agent of the danger to adopt a new strategy.
Our wolf had designs on the flock but chose to flee once the villagers responded to his attack. Similarly, a would-be thief who sees a
beware-of-dog sign in front of a house might skip it in favor of an
unprotected home.

Obviously, Hurricane Katrina was a naïve danger. It proceeded
according to the laws of nature, with no regard for human peril or
response. With the Yom Kippur War, it is not known whether the
original Arab mobilizations in May were the start of a long-term
strategy of deception or whether Israel's counter-mobilization de-
terred war the first time around by making it too costly for the at-
tackers. Israel's quick response in May made it impossible for
anyone to distinguish between a true alarm and a false one. Absent
any independent information about the situation, Israel recorded
the incident as a false alarm—as each of our brains is programmed
to do in similar circumstances. This situation, in which adaptive
danger wisely avoids confrontation, happens much more frequently
than does the deliberate false alarm set off by stupidity or malice.

Because security precautions tied to alert systems may cause the wolf, thief, or army to stop, the very success of the system may undermine its future effectiveness.

A third version of the "cry wolf" story is the most disturbing. Here, the wolf emerges from the forest but does not approach the flock. Instead, the wolf trots along the edge of the trees before disappearing back into the forest. The wolf's brief appearance does not cause the shepherd to sound the alarm. The next day, at the same time, the same wolf appears. He comes a little closer but again returns to the forest without doing any mischief. The shepherd remains alert. He decides that he will call out the village only if the wolf crosses the brook that is about halfway between the forest and his sheep. Day after day, the wolf comes and goes, slowly getting closer but never crossing the "red line." By now, our shepherd has become habituated to the wolf's behavior and "knows" that the wolf will always turn back into the forest.

Eventually, the wolf will be able to cross the brook and approach within striking distance of the sheep without causing the shepherd to call for help. The shepherd's perception of the threat is diminished by repeated mild exposure. The problem is the gradualism of the threat. Gradualism explains why people take up habits they know are bad for them. If we smoke a single cigarette, for example, nothing really bad happens. If we smoke another, nothing really bad happens. The consequences aren't likely to kick in for twenty to thirty years, when we develop lung cancer, emphysema, or another horrid disease. If danger is slow and gradual, the brain becomes used to it and begins to disregard it. To connect danger to the act of smoking, some parents, when they catch their kids in the act, immediately force them to smoke an entire pack. They know that smoking twenty cigarettes *will* make them sick. Suffering immediate painful (and temporary) consequences, the kids are more likely to put a stop to the behavior.

This disconnect between the act and the consequences is why the most dangerous types of drugs are the seemingly harmless ones. Few people start drug use by injecting heroin into their veins. People take milder drugs without suffering serious side effects. After a while, they move on to more serious drugs and begin to take them in more dangerous ways. Step by step, they become habituated to the act even as the wolf circles ever closer. Similar examples occur routinely. In the 1980s and 1990s, Americans lived with a mounting national debt and nothing bad seemed to happen. Some commentators even claimed that prosperous times proved that deficit spending meant little. The debt built, compounded by interest. Eventually, it created serious harm, worsening the impact of the great recession and greatly complicating efforts to end it. Repetitive but mild exposure to all kinds of danger disarms the precautions that sensible people would normally take.

FALSE PROMISES AND THREATS

Other forms of false alarms include false promises and false labels. In the heat of the moment, a parent might threaten a child with some dire consequence if the child *ever* repeats his or her current misbehavior. In many cases, the parent cannot or will not carry out the threat. The threatened punishment was too severe, it would spoil the upcoming weekend, or the other parent disagrees—who knows what. But this false alarm results in a major loss of credibility, undermining the parent's ability to control the child. Other promise-givers have similar problems. After failing to carry out a campaign pledge, a politician will have to offer up a great deal more before the next election, or nobody will listen.

Anyone in a position of power, whether it's someone with global power, such as a national leader, or someone with personal power, such as a parent or teacher, must be extremely careful when delivering promises or threats. They must be almost 100 percent certain that the promise or threat will be carried out. Otherwise, it is not worth the risk. A failure to act will be a blow to their credibility and therefore their cause.

False labeling is ever-present in our lives. Consider the notion of urgency. How many times is a secretary told that every memo, every appointment, every phone call, is "urgent"? A harried boss invariably says that the current task is the most pressing of the day. After a while, the meaning of urgency diminishes. Now the boss has to say, "This is super-urgent." Then, "This is super-super-urgent." If everything is urgent, then nothing is urgent. There is no way to prioritize. When working with colleagues, we should make a point of often saying, "This task is *not* urgent, take your time." Or, "This task can wait until you have done the first three." So if once in a long while, a matter *is* urgent, we know that colleagues will respond. And when we give them something time-critical to do, we should tell them what they can postpone in order to carry out the new task. Urgent must mean exceptional!

Intelligence agencies all over the world are the biggest culprits when it comes to false labeling. Everything becomes "top secret." Mislabeling occurs because of bureaucratic inertia or conservatism, the fear of accidentally releasing information that *does* turn out to be sensitive. Occasionally the reason is to cover up a mistake. If everything is top secret, however, nothing is. People deliberately leak information that they know should not have been classified, or they stop taking the categorization seriously. As a result, once in a while revelations occur that are highly damaging. If labels mean little, people will not honor them. Here, again, we see the impact of experience. Because of the frequency of the false alarm, because what should be unusual becomes usual, people stop paying attention.

In all these instances, prior false experience erodes credibility. In such circumstances, experience has taught the brain the lesson that labels cannot be trusted. However, this is the opposite of what the labels seek to achieve! The contradiction comes from a lack of understanding of how the brain works and of how credibility can actually be achieved.

CALIBRATING THE ALARMS

I have done a number of experiments to determine which features of a threat affect the power of false alarms. Two items turn out to be the main culprits: 1) the perceived probability of danger; and 2) the perceived severity of the danger. If an announcer says that a hurricane has an 80 percent chance of hitting Louisiana, and the storm veers away, the loss of credibility is much, much greater than if the announcer says there is a 15 to 20 percent chance. Perceived severity includes physical proximity to the danger as well as how soon it is supposed to happen. If a "red alert" occurs for a terrorist attack in our town—a severe and *imminent* risk of danger locally—and no attack occurs, the loss of credibility is much, much greater than if the alert had been for the lower "orange" or "yellow" level. Loss of belief in the system is higher if the reported risk is higher, so the highest warning stage must be reserved until we are very sure something is going to happen. The highest level of alert should never be called off.

Here is a contradiction. Usually the organization and the people who are personally responsible for safety tend to *upgrade* a threat to be absolutely sure that everyone takes it seriously. If an attack occurs, the warning system is validated. But if the attack does not materialize, the system loses credibility in proportion to the level of the warning. From a psychological perspective, *downgrading* a threat should be the default policy. Yet what bureaucrat wants to downgrade a threat only to have an attack occur? Especially if a lowering of the threat level itself encourages the attack. The United States abandoned its color-coded terrorist alert system nine years after 9/11 precisely because it proved to be meaningless and un-workable. The new alert system has only two levels: "elevated," if there is an indication of a terrorist attack but no specific informa-tion about the timing or location; and "imminent," if there is cred-ible information about an impending attack in a particular locale.

It's important to maintain the long-term credibility of our warn-ing systems. One way would be to minimize the stated probability initially and ratchet it up as the nature of the danger becomes clearer. As long as there is a reasonable chance it might not materialize, underplaying a threat is better than overplaying it. A parallel argu-ment exists for documents that are labeled urgent or top secret. Minimizing such descriptions, "trading down" our terminology as much as possible, will maintain the long-term legitimacy of the sys-tem. But the people in charge are concerned less with the long-term credibility of the system than they are with how citizens respond *today*.

These examples all illustrate the difficulty of dealing with false alarms. If we experience repeated false alarms, we are lulled to sleep. If we overstate threats, we are lulled to sleep. Imagine how this quandary might affect those who are in charge of emergency responses and military security. One argument is that there should be frequent rotation in these jobs. In order to properly evaluate all of the signs of danger and give a fresh, dispassionate appraisal of the latest threat, the people at the heart of the alert system need to be unbiased by previous exposure to threats that did not materialize. The worst thing for the people in these jobs to have is too much experience! The long-term credibility (and therefore functionality) of the system must also be protected. The people in charge should not overstate threats, even legitimate ones, but instead ensure an orderly step up in the alert status. There should be two distinct job positions. The first position would ensure that we correctly pick up on actual threats. The second would ensure that the populace continues to listen to warnings over time.

Decision makers in emergency response systems need protection against the public's reaction to false alarms. Consider the mayor of a low-lying township. If an earthquake occurs off the coast and she follows the regulations, she has to evacuate the town. But the chances for a tsunami are low. Elections are nearing and the constituents are still grumbling about the last evacuation, which turned out to be unnecessary. The next time the threat rears its head, the mayor decides not to order an evacuation. Of course, this is when the tsunami hits. In an electoral system, the person who "cries wolf" is held personally responsible for every false alarm. Leaders are highly motivated *not* to call the next one. This is what happened to Israeli Defense Minister Moshe Dayan, who was chastised for wasting resources when he authorized the general mobilization in May 1973. The result? He did not summon the military soon enough in October. People who have to make these difficult decisions need to be shielded from any negative consequences of the alert.

FALSE ALARMS HAPPEN TO EVERYONE, ALL THE TIME

Whether in work, politics, or our personal lives, we can all think of examples in which a false alarm caused us to disregard a later legitimate threat. It turns out that false alarms can even affect our lives at the cellular level. Our immune system is designed to fight any biological entity that appears to be not-of-our-own-body or otherwise harmful. In addition to attacking bacteria and viruses that have invaded the body, the immune system also attacks cancerous cells within the body. However, repeated exposure to harmless mutations of body cells can cause the immune system to tolerate similar malignant mutations in the future.

To overcome the danger of biological false alarms, we would have to develop medical techniques that cause our immune system to treat even innocent mutations as dangerous. This would, however, inevitably enhance the threat of autoimmune disease. There's a trade-off. To overcome the danger of false alarms in our individual lives, we need to force our brains to step out of the false-alarm trap. All that's required is a change in perspective. To avoid complacency, we should not ask the question, "Did it come true?" Instead, we should change our perspective by asking, "Can I afford to ignore the risk?"

It is better to develop a mindset to board up our houses and run for the hills—even unnecessarily—rather than suffer destruction if an alarm turns out *not* to be false. We also need to be alert to the gradual degradation of credibility that occurs in many relationships, when the disparity between our words and actions causes us to resort to ever more extreme measures. We need only the occasional word of praise or censure to achieve results, provided that our behavior is consistent with what we say. On the other hand, if our actions do not match our words, the brain picks up on the discrepancy quickly. The threat or promise loses impact.

It is almost impossible to ignore the false lessons of false alarms. Experience teaches us to reach the easiest and most reassuring conclusion rather than the correct one about potential dangers. This is the first important clue about the downside of experience. Unexamined experience teaches us to ignore danger signs. An inability to "unlearn" from experience entraps us in false security. But this is only the start when it comes to how experience can freeze our minds.

=== **LESSONS IN BRAINPOWER** ===

- It is difficult for us to unlearn something, especially if it gives us false comfort.
- A single false alarm reduces our reaction to subsequent alarms by as much as 50 percent. The more severe the warning, the greater the negative impact of the false alarm.
- Our perception of threat is diminished by repeated mild exposure.
- Punishing people for sounding false alarms makes it less likely that they will warn people the next time—when the danger might be real.
- Our tendency to be lulled to sleep by false alarms is proof that experience often teaches us the wrong lessons.

THREE

The Many Dangers of Experience

For most of humanity's existence, reliance on experience has been a good thing. It has become a bad thing primarily because the speed of cultural evolution has outstripped the speed of biological evolution. For countless millennia, most of our forebears' energy and brainpower were expended in survival. All they needed to know was how to avoid predators and find enough food for themselves. These skills were relatively specific and concrete and could be transferred to new environments. The requirements of a hunter-gatherer in New Guinea were not, after all, much different than the requirements for one in Africa or Europe. Even after the shift to agriculture, societies changed very little over hundreds or even thousands of years. Early humans lived difficult and dangerous lives, but their lives were—nonetheless—relatively stable. Survival in this kind of world favored "once-and-for-all learning," in the words of John Pfeiffer. Early and rapid learning settled into relatively fixed actions and attitudes that served people admirably for the entirety of their short lives.

All learning, in fact, is based on the assumption of stability. Our environment must remain consistent long enough for us to learn how to cope with it and predict and prepare for the future. When we successfully predict the correct solution to a situation based on what was effective in the past, we learn that experience works. (Biologically, the humans who relied on experience survived longer and reproduced more, thereby bringing this trait forward in our genes.) Reliance on experience brings with it a double whammy. It does work, most of the time. But because experience requires stability, it causes us to *expect* stability. Successful learning, or habit formation, enhances our belief in a stable world. And that's where we get into trouble.

As humans shifted from agrarian societies to urban ones, as technological progress began to accelerate, as unruly democracies supplanted traditional kingships, and as the economies of nations became ever more interconnected, many measures of quality of life increased—but stability plummeted. The instability of the modern world has reduced our ability to accurately predict the future, making adjustment difficult and reliance on experience problematic. What happens to behavior that was successfully employed for years when it is challenged by new circumstances? How can we effectively adjust to environments that have become moving targets? How does a septuagenarian who grew up before television comprehend today's world of instant and nonstop digital communication?

In a changing world, it is our ability to unlearn that will determine our ability to survive, adapt, and move forward.

Having experience is far less important than being able to abandon experience when circumstances require it. Unlearning experience (the "extinction of learned behavior") is quite difficult. When the original learning involves the avoidance of something painful or dangerous, extinction becomes almost impossible to achieve. A classic example is the child who suffers a horrible fright or injury because of a vicious dog. The child avoids going anywhere near the dog's house—even years later, long after the dog has likely died—and reacts with extreme fear to the friendliest of dogs. Even into adulthood, he or she may still believe that avoidance is the only solution to the problem. This prewired reaction has significant survival value, particularly if the beast being avoided is a lion from the savannah instead of a dog from the neighbor's yard. Yet this story illustrates the main difficulty with this kind of behavior. The same actions that protect us from confronting a frightening situation also

EMOTIONAL SECURITY LEADS TO COGNITIVE SECURITY

Early and rapid learning is a hallmark of all primates, particularly humans. Early emotional attachment between mother and infant is critical to healthy personality development. Human infants share with other primates the need for secure attachments as a prerequisite for effective exploration of their environment. Lacking the emotional security provided by the mother, the infant is unwilling to undertake the exploration needed to learn the necessary skills to adjust to life's challenges. The infant is too anxious to attend to the world around it.

Research with primates provides dramatic evidence of the importance of solid infant-mother attachment. Infant rhesus monkeys taken from their mothers and raised by surrogates react to novelty with screams of pain as if they were being tortured. Monkeys separated from their mothers for as few as six days suffer negative aftereffects to novelty more than two years later. Reactions to novel stimuli are such a sensitive index to emotional disturbance that the "stranger situation"—how a child behaves when left alone with a stranger—is used as an experimental measure of emotional security. The level of a child's distress relates directly to his or her level of emotional insecurity. Early emotional learning, perhaps even more than other types of learning, is particularly resistant to subsequent extinction.

Though psychological literature focuses on "mother-infant" bonds, in actuality babies in traditional societies have a wide interaction with other (usually female) adults, "aunties" in various guises. Children have the capacity, and likely the need, for wide intimacies with other adults, siblings, and cousins. Modern urban life, particularly in the middle classes, has isolated the mother and child from the rest of society. Throughout most of human history, the opportunity to form wider associations through time spent with peers and the extended family relieved some of the pressure of an exclusive mother-infant relationship. The overwhelming predominance of the mother may significantly cripple the child's ability to form good social relationships with a wide range of different people. A doting mother may inadvertently stunt her child's emotional growth and hamper his or her ability to explore the world—always a risky enterprise, even for the most emotionally secure.

Most people would think of this as an emotional problem, but it is a cognitive one, too. Insecurity tremendously reduces the child's level of curiosity and exploration, which are major elements in cognitive development. There are also lifelong repercussions on how the person will approach exploration and risk. Along with every emotional problem is an associated cognitive problem. In this case, it is another example in which experience teaches the brain the wrong lesson. Or at least, it has taught the brain a lesson that no responsible parent wants to teach: that children lack the strength to face the world on their own.

prevent us from finding out whether that situation still exists. In the absence of "reality testing," a person has no chance to unlearn workable but immature solutions.

FALLING INTO (BAD) HABITS

Automatic information processing and automatic behavior has many advantages. As we learn a new skill, the brain becomes increasingly efficient. The experienced reader does not have to decode each letter separately and combine them into words, as a beginner does. Automatic word recognition not only saves valuable time and energy, but also frees us to attend to the meaning of the text, rather than its decoding. Comprehension increases. We can drive a car beyond the speed of thought because we learn the skill so well that it becomes automatic. It is only when we are driving in difficult and unfamiliar conditions—for instance, in a country where the traffic is on the opposite side of the road—that we have to consciously consider our actions. We rarely think about what it takes to balance ourselves on a bicycle, no matter how long it has been since we last rode one.

Few behaviors are fully automatic, however. Standing isn't, as witnessed by our inability to sleep upright. And walking is not entirely automatic, either. If we doubt that it requires our attention, we can take a friend out for a leisurely stroll and try the following experiment: As we walk, we tell our friend something that we know is of great personal interest to him. As the meaning of our words absorbs his attention, he will not have enough cognitive resources left over for walking. He will probably stop in his tracks. If the information is dramatic or painful, he may actually need to lean on something, or sit down. We have all seen someone become immobilized by extremely good or bad news. This effect is primarily caused by the brain's preoccupation with the news, augmented in the case of catastrophic news by shock, which constricts the blood supply to the limbs.

As long as any behavior is semiautomatic, we have the opportunity to intervene and change it. This is important, because automaticity, despite being efficient and often useful, precludes innovation and change. It is inappropriate in situations that are different enough from past situations to require new thinking. Our goal should be to slow our actions and decisions down before they become automatic. Fatigue can slow cognitive processes, enabling new ideas to creep in, which is why running, biking, and other physical exercise often "clears the cobwebs" after a morning in the office. The combination of increased blood flow and weariness opens the brain to new concepts. (Even something like a cold can lead to fresh thinking, by slowing us down but not otherwise rendering us inoperative.) *Anything* that slows information processing can help us overcome automaticity. The nature of automaticity is speed. From the moment it begins to the moment it ends, we have no opportunity to interfere and change the process.

Automaticity can also be affected by state-dependent learning. We tend to remember things best while we're in the same physical and mental state as when we first learned them. This phenomenon can lead to curious results. A group of people was divided into two teams. One team was given a glass of whiskey; the other remained sober. Both teams were given a list of words to memorize. As expected, the sober group did better than the whiskey group. The next day the whiskey group was tested again. The group was divided into two teams, one that had *another* drink of whiskey and one that remained sober. *The team that drank whiskey the second day did better than the team that stayed sober.* Because they first learned the words while slightly inebriated, they did better when slightly inebriated the next time. Repeating the initial context in which the learning occurred led to better memory than a change of context . . . even though the change (sobriety) should have improved cognitive function.

Conversely, changing the state in which we learned something can be used to break automaticity. Some companies are famous for having brainstorming sessions in hallways and stairwells. The purpose is to remove people from the context in which they ordinarily think. A change in environment is also why teams go on retreats, to create a new physical and mental state in which fresh thought is stimulated. This is also why doing business on a golf course is not necessarily a wastrel's activity, provided that the golf course represents a *change* and is not the usual state in which work is carried out.

We should deliberately seek out not just new physical states but also new mental states when we are facing important issues. One way to encourage fresh thought is to develop a list of questions designed to challenge our basic assumptions about the situation before us. The crucial issue is to try to crack the brain's belief that "similar is identical," which puts us on the fast track to repeating earlier behaviors even if the similarity does not run true. If we made money by buying a house in the 1980s, and again in the 1990s, experience teaches us that we should be able to buy another house in the 2000s and "flip it" for a profit. This nationwide mindset created the U.S. housing boom—and bust. Rather than accepting the unspoken assumption that housing prices will always rise, we might ask what has changed in the economy after a decade, or whether any market has *ever* continued to rise unabashedly year after year.

The best way to challenge our assumptions is to ask what other set of circumstances might explain the situation besides the ones we presuppose. Are we, for example, at the back end of a wave in which other flippers have artificially driven up housing prices? Another way to avoid the trap of automaticity is to ask trusted friends—preferably ones with diverse backgrounds—for their perspectives in order to see the situation in a new light. Brainstorming works best when participants include people with a variety of experiences, skills, and responsibilities—people who bring their unique frames of reference to the table.

All of these solutions assume that we are not already locked into automatic behavior. Just as the best person to build an expert system is not an expert (who is unable to articulate how she does what she does) but rather a skilled but not expert practitioner (who still is able to describe what he does and the steps involved), the best person to deal with change is someone who is not on full automatic pilot.

When our behaviors are fully automatic, we are out of luck. Neurotic behavior is an extreme example, but we are all capable of falling into harmful patterns of behavior. Consider the family dynamic in which a parent and teen argue over the teen's curfew. The parent invariably says that the teen is being irresponsible. The teen invariably says that the parent is trying to control her life. Both feel provoked, and that provocation leads to inflexible responses. They argue repeatedly, almost from a script, embodying the metaphor of the "broken record." Each is having more of an internal monologue than an external dialogue.

Imagine that this same parent and child are having a similar argument over control issues, except now the parent is sixty and the child is thirty-five. Or think of a couple long divorced who fall into the same arguments they suffered decades before in their marriage. Unfortunately, automatic behaviors in our personal relationships are hard to escape, because they begin so early and run so deep. We are often imprisoned in a dense web of automaticity. Our habitual reactions to our nagging parents may not qualify as neurosis, but they are bad for us and for those around us. Such ingrained patterns explain why family counseling often focuses on reframing issues in ways that encourage both sides to consider a new point of view.

DESCENDING INTO RIGIDITY AND FIXATION

The historic and prehistoric need of humans to learn early and rapidly before settling into a routine may be a major reason we fall so easily into rigidity of thought and behavior. The forceful, often devastating grip of the past over human affairs is evident in many psychological illnesses. Each school of psychotherapy has its own way of describing mental issues, but they all agree that neurotics are tied to the past, out of touch with the present or future, and "wrecked by [their] rigidity" (Freud's phrase). Vast clinical evidence of rigidity among neurotics and psychotics receives support from experimental studies as well. Neurotics exhibit higher levels of rigidity than psychotics, and both have higher levels than other people.

Whatever form it takes, psychotherapy seeks to treat mental and emotional problems by loosening the grip of these rigid attitudes. Traditional psychotherapy assumes that by opening up childhood issues within the accepting atmosphere of the therapeutic session, people can begin to unfreeze behavior patterns that have been entrenched for years. Behavior modification seeks to change the repetitive behavior itself, resolving the problem from the outside in by rewiring the compulsion. And positive psychology tries to help a person build a new, positive self-image of him- or herself by building upon the person's strengths and positive experiences and rendering ancient trauma moot. Rigid behavior patterns are often defensive in nature, so they do not go easily, whatever the approach. Mental health professionals are aware of the need to effectively deal with resistance to the treatment itself. What psychotherapy attempts to do is nothing short of de-automatization of behavior. This is extremely difficult because it is hard to slow deeply rooted emotional and psychological reactions enough that a person will open up to new responses.

Irrespective of the problem at hand, and across the spectrum of therapies, the task of un-fixating a troubled mind remains a gargantuan challenge. The reason is obvious: We are basically a conservative lot, and any attempt at change is bound to run into major problems. *This conservatism and our overreliance on experience not only create issues with our behaviors and decisions but also pose a threat to the underlying health of the brain.* Reliance on experience precludes significant mental effort and exposure to novelty, both of which are needed to stimulate the brain. Going the traditional way, without thinking, is one of the main obstacles to cognitive health.

THE GREATEST DANGER OF EXPERIENCE

As with "expert," the root of "experience" is "experiri," a Latin word meaning "to try out." People with a lot of experience should be willing to try new things, as their knowledge should open them to new possibilities. However, just as experts do not routinely try new things—but unconsciously pull answers from a vast cognitive database of things tried before—so too do highly experienced people tend to fall into the habits of the past. Relying on experience is fast and efficient, and it can provide a useful shortcut for decision making. But it comes at a price. When we rely on experience, we risk solving today's problems with yesterday's solutions. We apply past patterns to the future. (Think of the townspeople who ignored the shepherd boy after his first false alarm.) Rather than call upon its amazing creativity, we too often use our brain as nothing more than a huge storage bin of precedents.

Because "close is good enough," we need not think afresh. We need not examine new data or evaluate new circumstances. Our brain fills in the blanks for us. This is the main problem with elderly people. No matter what circumstances confront them today, they have seen, heard, and dealt with so many situations in their lives that they are bound to have faced something similar before. *Senior citizens have too much experience.* This comment may sound ironic, but experience can be detrimental when it leads to an automated response to a new situation. This happens to me as much as to anyone. A student will come in with a fresh new topic for a research paper or dissertation. I will suggest several ideas for their project. The ideas are new to the student, but they are not new to me. They come from my data vault without me even being aware of it. The same thing happens with other matters as well. When dealing with family problems, it is easy to reach back for a solution that suited the 1950s or 1970s but may not be appropriate today. Think of the stories our elders tell us, starting "When I was a young man . . ." or "Back when I was working at the . . ." Sometimes these stories impart wisdom, but more often than not they are stereotyped responses that may cause the speaker's adult children or teenage grandchildren to roll their eyes. These stories are told constantly, no matter how peripherally they relate to the situation at hand.

This kind of reflexive response is part of the human predisposition to learn early and quickly and then fall into a habitual manner of thought. This behavior is consistent with earlier, simpler, and often more dangerous times. Learning survival skills quickly and then relying on them for life was advantageous for early humans. But in the modern world, in which change rather than stability is the order of the day, reliance on experience is often inappropriate. Even the best of us struggle throughout our lives with the habituation of experience. We struggle to unlearn things that were once useful and are now holding us back.

Drifting into intellectual and emotional rigidity, we too often draw the wrong lessons from life. For some of us, emotional or physical trauma occurs so early that we become locked into a limited pattern of behavior that can stunt our emotional growth or make us totally dysfunctional. The underlying theme of all of these examples is the speed with which humans descend into automaticity. Automaticity is the opposite of maximum brainpower. Precisely because of its attention-free speed, automaticity creates problems when we are faced with new situations and important changes. The question we must continually confront is whether, in a particular situation, the brain draws upon experience because it summons up valuable learning or because pulling a quick answer from the data bank is easier than applying fresh deliberation.

Habit, says psychologist William James, is the fly-wheel of society, its most precious conservative agent. It holds the miner in his darkness and keeps the poor from rising up. So bound by habit are we, he says, that the characteristic mindset of each profession becomes visible by a person's twenties. We constantly fight the battle of life upon the lines imposed by (our personal) traditions and routines; that is, by our experience. Rather than having experience *inform* our choices, too often experience *defines* our choices. Experience is our best teacher, unless we give it too much heed. *Unlearning old habits* is the real key to learning!

For senior citizens, this problem is particularly vexing. The number one priority of the elderly should be to continually challenge their brains in ways that are constructive and effortful. Experience can halt the development of brainpower. Relying on precedents is good for many decisions in life, but it is not for our cognitive sustenance. The danger of experience is not merely that it can betray us into the wrong answer. The greater jeopardy is that too great a reliance on experience will stop the brain from thinking—from doing work. When experience forecloses significant mental effort, brainpower narrows and cognitive decline sets in. For anyone, at any age.

===== LESSONS IN BRAINPOWER =====

- We learn early and quickly but then tend to settle into relatively fixed attitudes for the rest of our lives.
- For experience to work, our lives must remain more or less the same—a practical impossibility in today's ever-changing world. Thus, it is our ability to *unlearn,* not learn, that will determine our success.
- Because our brains so readily fill in the blanks, we run the risk of filling them in with old data that no longer applies to the situation at hand.
- The elderly's reliance on experience precludes mental effort and exposure to novelty, both of which are needed to stimulate the brain.
- Experience is one of the main obstacles to cognitive health.

FOUR

Disordered Thought or Genius?

Imagine that, when we speak of the animal that ate the flowers in our garden, no one understands what we're talking about because we use the names of various animals interchangeably. Imagine that our mention of gardening yesterday reminds us of paying bills today and the thought of paying bills today jumps our brain to the trip we need to make to the bank tomorrow and the thought of the bank reminds us that we also need to go to the grocery store next to the bank. As we describe these thoughts, a friend tells us to quit beating around the bush and get to the point. We are confused because we are in an office, nowhere near a bush, but the thought of a bush launches us again into thoughts of gardening and the creature that ate our flowers. . . .

Welcome to the world of schizophrenia.

Schizophrenia is a cognitive disorder that causes people to perceive reality far differently than most others do. Common symptoms are disorganized thought and language, the hearing of voices, paranoia, and withdrawal from society. Brain scans show that, compared to other people, schizophrenics have less activation of the frontal lobes, which provide coordination and executive control over other brain functions. Some parts of the brain are more active, though the overall pattern of activity is more diffuse and scattered than typical.

Schizophrenia has so many variations that a number of researchers consider it to be several related disorders rather than a single major disorder. The focus here is what is generally called "disorganized schizophrenia" or "formal thought disorder." The "disorganization" of the schizophrenic provides a window into the way all of us learn. The key is "connections." If schizophrenics are on the extreme end of the spectrum in connecting things, the ability to relate "A" to "B" is, nonetheless, at the heart of learning. The capacity to associate things that are close is necessary for comprehension and for managing everything that we do. The difference between "thought disorder" and "brilliance" turns out to be a matter of degree.

DERAILING THE TRAIN OF THOUGHT

The mental processes of people with disorganized schizophrenia can be difficult to follow. The phrase "knight's move" has been used to describe their thought processes. Their logic seems to simultaneously jump one forward and two sideways. One thought is often derailed by another and loose associations can lead to strange leaps in logic. Schizophrenics also tend to jump to conclusions, particularly with regard to negative stimuli, and they may obsessively focus on potential threats. They often hear voices—sometimes talking to them, sometimes giving them orders, sometimes talking to one another. Speech difficulties range from excessive rhyming to circumlocution to repetition of words and phrases to "word salad"—coherent words strung together in seemingly incoherent ways. Suffering from overgeneralization and excessive linkages, the language of schizophrenics becomes unintelligible.

The problem is not that schizophrenics cannot connect the dots. It is that they connect too many dots in too many different ways. They lack the ability to block distracting thoughts—something the rest of us can do in our conscious minds. For most of us, the way we think silently is fundamentally different from the way we talk—and even the way we verbalize in our minds. In our silent thoughts, anything goes. We have no need to think systematically, and we don't. An interior or exterior monologue immediately imposes discipline on the mental process. We need to organize our thoughts to stay on track, either to solve problems, make plans, or complete tasks. Schizophrenics talk the way the rest of us think silently, without any focus or organization.

Combined, the result is that schizophrenics see connections among a flurry of thoughts that seem unrelated to other folks. As in the opening scenario, they may consider all four-legged creatures to be interchangeable; thus, they might use the words "giraffe," "cow," "pig," and "camel" to describe the same animal. They might connect events by time, place, or some other association that's less than obvious. Their flow of logic might tie together everything that stems from, or results in, a certain emotion or state of mind. Thus, a book on art history, a meal of Mexican food, a football game, and a conversation with a cousin might be as tightly and logically connected in their minds as the beginning, middle, and end of a one-topic story is to the rest of us.

Freud viewed our unconscious as operating via "primary processes," which mainly manifest themselves as images welling up without chronological sequence, order, causality, or logic. The raw stuff of the brain, if you will. Our consciousness applies "secondary processes" to organize, order, and provide causality to these uncooked ingredients. Schizophrenics have the primary processes but few, if any, of the secondary ones.

Non-schizophrenics experience these primary processes in their dream life, Freud's "royal road" to the unconscious. In dreams, meaning is often hidden in symbolization, condensation, and displacement. Contrary to popular belief, determining the symbolism of dreams is usually straightforward and relatively universal. Whole catalogs exist on the meanings of common dreams, with bountiful case studies that seem to validate the interpretations. A dream of falling usually represents anxiety or uncertainty about some event, for example, and a dream of flying usually represents a sense of accomplishment and power. Condensation and displacement obscure the central idea that's preoccupying the mind. For example, condensation can make one thing of multiple concerns; worries about sev-

eral people or events may coalesce into a single threatening figure in
a dream. A simple instance of displacement involves Freud himself,
who once dreamed of vanquishing a rival with a "piercing look."
On reflection, he realized that the dream involved an experience in
which his mentor, Ernest Brücke, had given him a harsh glare and a
dressing down for reporting late to his teaching duties. Freud's
dream displaced the facts to lessen the embarrassment of his come-
uppance.

Understanding the mental processes behind dreams helped Freud
frame his approach to analysis, in which he attempted to reach re-
pressed memories by having the patient lie quietly on a couch in a
dark, quiet room and freely associate ideas. The setting was intended to re-create aspects of sleep in an effort to loosen the control
of the conscious (ego) over the unconscious (id). Freud's actual interpretations of dreams, as well as some of his analyses of his patients' mental problems, have been criticized for a number of
reasons. What is important here is his evaluation of how the conscious often censors the unconscious and how even the unconscious
may be masking a "forbidden" idea. A "forbidden" idea is not necessarily one that is taboo for cultural or ethical reasons. It is any
idea that is out of the ordinary—out of the usual mental rut. Making unusual connections is how the unconscious can free itself from
censorship. The freeing of the mind to make new and interesting
connections is what ties together disordered mental states, dreams,
and creativity.

What are dreams to us may well be the typical conscious state of
schizophrenics. Through their speech, we can directly observe the
seething cauldron of disorganized cognition in their thoughts, in
which images dominate over logic. Yet that troubled unconscious
can also be a font of creativity. John Nash, the mathematician whose
life was chronicled in the book and movie *A Beautiful Mind*, suffered from paranoid schizophrenia, but he also developed Nobel
Prize–winning game theory that could be applied to fields as diverse
as economics, warfare, and evolution. He was also one of the first
to reject traditional psychiatric treatment for his condition, ultimately learning (he said) to ignore his delusions.

NEW MEANINGS FROM STRANGE CONNECTIONS

If schizophrenia is marked by a compulsive excess of loose connections, some of the most creative thought also comes from improbable connections. To paraphrase Marvin Minsky, who cofounded the artificial intelligence lab at MIT, a thing with just one meaning has scarcely any meaning at all. An idea that chugs along in only one specific direction will often lead to a dead end and rigidity of thought. We know this intuitively when we speak negatively of someone with a "one-track mind." The idea "buying a house," for instance, is unlikely to bring up one discrete idea. For most of us, it would bring up thoughts about home styles, paint colors, interior design, mortgage costs, potential repairs, things we liked and disliked about houses in the past, good and bad locations, and so on. When an initial thought has multiple meanings, we have the opportunity to turn over in our minds many related ideas and tangential notions and consider a number of alternatives, which is the very essence of thinking. Nash, our experts, and other highly creative people are those who see unique perspectives among multiple potential meanings that the rest of us miss. Sometimes the line between brilliance and disordered thought is paper thin: Shakespeare is nearly as guilty of excessive punning as many schizophrenics, and the immoderate rhyming associated with schizophrenia would be right at home at any contemporary poetry slam. Indeed, the brain's ability to treat as "identical" two things that are distantly connected is the basis for our ability to create and enjoy poetry, jokes, and other forms of wordplay and to solve certain kinds of math problems.

In the Renaissance, poetry was a logical construction in which images helped make the central argument more concrete. In "Valediction Forbidding Mourning," John Donne compares two souls to a protractor, the mechanical device used to draw a circle. One soul is the "fix'd foot"; the other moves about it. No matter how they are pulled apart, they remain as one and they eventually end up together. The extremity of the contrast (two souls = one protractor) is both the challenge of the poem and the pleasure of it. Shakespeare

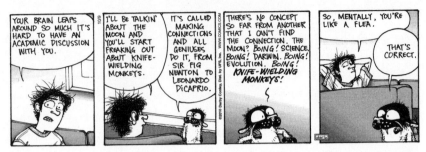

Figure 4-1. Making unexpected connections is the hallmark of individuals who are either brilliant or mentally troubled, and Bucky the cartoon cat illustrates how fine the line can be between genius and insanity. *(GET FUZZY © 2010 Darby Conley. Reprinted by permission of Universal Uclick for UFS. All rights reserved.)*

provides a litany of ways in which his love is unlike all of the standard comparisons to the sun, roses, perfume, music, and goddesses. His conclusion, that he thinks his love as rare as any woman "belied with false compare," contains multiple verbal twists. After first working through the many standard metaphors (sun = bright face and eyes, roses = red cheeks and lips, etc.), we must throw away the comparisons as being trite next to a real human being.

One trend in modern poetry has been the stripping away of this "progression by argument" style. In its place many poets are using exposition by image. The shower of arrows fired into the air by poet Philip Larkin comes down as "gentle rain." Larkin does not give us a neat and logical conclusion through artful argument. Instead, arrows-into-rain is used as a metaphor for the superficiality and ennui of life in postwar England. The underlying theme emerges through the linkage of images, many of them less than obvious— not unlike schizophrenia. As in Samuel Beckett's plays, which over time shrink in action and dialogue, an image-only approach can become so thin that the reader must supply most, if not all, of the interpretation—and sense. The mind must fill in the blanks. William Carlos Williams's most famous poem, "The Red Wheelbarrow," does little more than state the existence of a farm implement. It is hard to know whether it represents Zen-like profundity or is a parody of the type.

Poets try to expand our ability to associate different aspects of the world. In so doing, they reveal the underlying connectedness of life. By juxtaposing the familiar with the horrific, some poets also force us to face uncomfortable truths that we as a civilization would rather forget. Somewhere between most of us unimaginative people and schizophrenics lies the edgy chaos of creativity, where the roiling brain makes connections that are broader than normal but still comprehensible, where abstract symbols create associations that resonate with our peers, and where new insights about the world are born. However much the conscious brain may organize these connections, they begin with images and symbols.

Many of history's greatest thinkers have said their best ideas came to them in dreams, when their conscious controls were weakened. Among such people are the French mathematician Henri Poincaré, the French philosopher René Descartes, and the British author Robert Louis Stevenson. Awakened by a loud noise, the mathematician Jacques Hadamard had the solution to a difficult problem instantly in his mind—one that was different from any he was pursuing. Hadamard, in fact, said that most of his solutions came to him as images rather than as conscious thoughts; after surveying other scientists, he found that the same was true for many of them. The German chemist August Kekulé is famous for saying that he developed the structure of benzene from a dream in which he saw a snake eating its tail—the image of Ouroboros, an ancient symbol for the cycle of life.

These creative linkages come from the same brain biology that seeks solutions that require minimal effort. For creativity to happen, "mistakes" must be made. To do good, nature must err. Without genetic mutations, which are nothing more than biological errors, we would still be amoeba in the Earth's primordial ooze. Most of the time, the brain makes reasonable connections between events. A few times, it makes unreasonable connections. Rarely, it makes improbable connections that turn out to be right in unexpected ways. The "error" turns out to be more efficient than the original. When the brain associates concepts that turn out to be connected on a deep level, we develop new solutions and invent new things. On both the biological and mental level, creativity is perhaps primarily a good mistake, an association of unlikely items that leads to a positive result.

Like poems, jokes use wordplay to give an ordinary situation an unexpected twist. Sometimes the humor derives from the situation and sometimes from puns or similar verbal ploys. A man once bought a twenty-four-piece jigsaw puzzle. It took hard work, but he was proud to finish in several weeks because the label on the box said "From two to four years." Another man succeeded in stealing several valuable paintings from a museum in Paris, but he was captured nearby when his large vehicle ran out of fuel. He cited poverty as the reason for his failure: "I had no Monet to buy Degas to make the Van Gogh." Then there was the meeting between the actors Arnold Schwarzenegger and Tom Cruise in which Arnold wanted Tom to play opposite him in a movie about composers: "You'll be Mozart. I'll be Bach." (Fans of *The Terminator* movie will understand this last one.)

In jokes, as in poetry, we must notice the discrepancy between the actual versus the perceived situation or be able to understand the multiple senses being applied to a single set of words. We must see how something is simultaneously both the same and different. Humor comes from our ability to read the meaning correctly while recognizing how the meaning might be misconstrued. This ability presupposes that somewhere there exist people who do *not* see the absurdity, like the Englishman who misunderstood *A Modest Proposal*, Jonathan Swift's bitter satire on social injustice. Reading that Londoners eased the burden of the Irish poor by eating Irish children, the gentleman slammed the book shut and declared, "I don't believe a word of it!" The fun of a double entendre (double intention) comes from our ability to simultaneously read both the innocent and the naughty intent. However, a double entendre can also enrich the meaning of serious works, as when Jesus calls Peter "the rock on which the church stands," punning on his disciple's name, Peter, and on the Greek word for "rock," *petras*.

We think of humor as "light," but it is emblematic of the deep insights that come in all creative endeavors when we connect the normally unconnected. It is the unexpected connections that give us the pleasure of solving a math puzzle, a riddle, a poem, or a joke. Every time we make idiomatic jumps in the brain, we resolve the stress of uncertainty (how are her eyes like the sea?) and we get a shot of dopamine as a reward for the solution (her eyes are green, they have unplumbed depths, and at times they are cold and stormy). Freud would add that part of the delight is that the often non-logical solutions represent a victory of the unconscious in circumventing the editing, control, and censorship of our logical conscious brain.

IMPRECISION IS THE BASIS FOR LEARNING

Excessive connections are examples of the "Von Domarus principle," a concept developed by psychiatrist Eilhard von Domarus to describe the mental processes of schizophrenics. Technically, schizophrenics are guilty of the fallacy of the undistributed middle, the logic of which is: All C are A; all D are A; therefore, all C are D. Thus, all giraffes are pigs because both have four feet. However, it does not appear to be a flaw in logic that leads to this conclusion; rather, the raw processing power of the unconscious slams together two somewhat alike items and fuses them into one. The conscious, thoughtful brain is unable to wrest them apart.

Though schizophrenics are extreme examples, the Von Domarus principle is actually at the heart of how everyone learns. The principle explains much about creativity in general, because learning requires the linking of similar concepts, and because the brain has the ability to take information from one situation and apply it to another. There *are* many useful similarities among four-legged animals. Mammals range in size from the one-inch (thirty-mm) bumblebee bat to the one-hundred-foot (thirty-meter) blue whale, yet they have many shared traits. Among the 5,400 mammalian species, it happens that giraffes, cows, pigs, and camels are, in fact, closely related. They share a common ancestor, they are physiologically similar, and they are all pack animals. If we understand the behavior of one species, we will have a good handle on the behavior of others. We *can* envision a single word to encompass all such creatures. That word is "ungulate." Our entire scientific classification of living creatures is based on broader and broader categories, many of them describing relationships that are not apparent to the layperson. What immediate similarities do we see between hippopotami and whales, for instance? DNA testing shows that hippos are more closely related to whales than to the land animals they physically resemble.

Our brain's ability to associate things that are "close" is not only the way we develop broad concepts and build our knowledge but also the way we make sense of the world on a daily basis. Cognitively, "close" must be "equal" in the real world. Otherwise, every time we saw the face of a loved one from a different angle, or in a different light, we would think we were seeing someone new. Every sunrise would bring us into new and confusing terrain; when passing clouds threw shadows across the land, the world would change again. Every differently sized triangle, rectangle, and square would be unique from all others. We could not recognize that "$a^2 + b^2 = c^2$" is the same formula as "$x^2 + y^2 = z^2$" or that "apple" and "APPLE" describe the same fruit. Every single thing and every single action would be unique and unrelatable to every other thing and action, for no two situations are ever exactly the same. Every moment would be miraculously new and frustratingly pointless. To keep the world from becoming a nightmare jumble of ever-new and ever-changing stimuli, we must simplify it through approximation. *The only way we can learn* is by the brain treating "similar" to mean "identical." Otherwise, the brain could never perceive relationships or discern trends.

The "close is good enough" approach is successful with many problems in our world, especially routine matters we see over and over, and it is also the source of creative thought and wordplay. But with every yin comes a yang. In an eerie parallel with the way expertise can slide into excessive reliance on experience, our tendency to make "similar" mean "identical" can take us from imaginative mental play to mental rigidity, as we will shortly see.

===== **LESSONS IN BRAINPOWER** =====

- Perceiving unity among similar ideas and objects is the only way we can comprehend reality amid billions of conflicting sensory inputs. It is how we make sense of the world.
- "Close is good enough" is a fundamental tendency of the brain.
- Our consciousness seeks to control or mask "forbidden ideas." Though this "editorial control" protects us from threatening or taboo subjects, it also tends to quash unusual ideas—anything out of the ordinary. Loosening the grip of the conscious mind can free the unconscious to make new, interesting, and useful connections—the essence of creativity.

FIVE

Don't Be Blind: Getting the Brain to See Afresh

Consider the hungry rat. There are two levers in its cage. One dispenses food every time it is pressed. The other dispenses food only 20 percent of the time. If the rat stumbles upon the 20-percent lever first, it will probably never investigate the other lever. When it finds a food source, it stops exploring. This behavior is prewired, part of the survival instinct. If something works, look no further. Do not waste additional energy on potentially better solutions, because they may not exist. Indeed, a continued search may cause us to lose what food we have already found.

Consider two hungry rats. One finds the 100-percent lever. The other finds the 20-percent lever. Now, both levers stop working. The rat that always received food and now receives nothing will very quickly begin to look elsewhere because going from "always" to "never" is a clear change of the rules. The rat who received food only once in every five tries, however, will go on pressing the lever for days, perhaps even weeks, before recognizing the change. Irregular reinforcement causes the brain to take longer to discover that a rule has changed.

Behaviors learned by partial and inconsistent reinforcement are exceedingly difficult to extinguish. The only place we can get consistent reinforcement to our behavior is in the lab. In real life, we seldom receive equal and regular reinforcement. We get just enough reinforcement for our old habits of thought to preclude fresh thinking. As a result, we default to old behaviors until we have an overwhelming and consistent amount of evidence of the need for change. Such evidence seldom presents itself until it is too late. If the rat is fed more or less randomly on a slowly increasing basis—receiving a pellet (say) once every three, twenty, seventy, one hundred tries, etc.—it will starve before it stops pressing the bar. Our basic conservatism comes from *satisfycing,* a psychological term that means we stop searching when we find a solution that is good enough. Satisfycing, together with partial reinforcement of seemingly "good enough" solutions, leads to mental rigidity. This all-pervasive danger even extends to how we view other people. Not only are we likely to stereotype others based on "tribal" characteristics—race, religion, gender, nationality, politics, etc.—but, as previously discussed, we face the danger of developing inflexibility in our daily interactions with our loved ones.

Though the Von Domarus principle was developed to explain the mental workings of schizophrenics, even "regular folks" rely excessively on unhelpful connections. In performing uncounted and complex physical, logical, and emotional calculations every second, the brain tries to conserve effort and to speed up its response time. Rather than working harder, it tries to work smarter. And that sometimes makes us dumb. Making connections with previous experience is the fastest way to avoid effort and create shortcuts, so the brain will often make the easiest connections rather than the best ones. The "close is good enough" process that enables us to learn and build a knowledge base becomes corrupted into satisfycing—doing just enough to get by, to find a solution that is less than optimal.

OUR COMMON ASSOCIATIONS

Mental rigidity can be seen in something as simple as the traditional word association test. When one person presents a word such as "black," the other person responds with the first word that comes to mind: invariably, "white." Human thought patterns are so consistent that entire books have been published presenting the normal response and the statistical distribution for common word associations. These associations run so deep that television shows such as the *Match Game, Hollywood Squares,* and *Family Feud* have aired for twenty or more years on the premise that contestants can match answers with celebrities, audiences, or the general public. Word association games are also popular online.

All commonly used words have a stereotypical response. On one word association test compiled from a hundred subjects, the word "down" elicited "up" about a third of the time; "dog" led to "cat" more than half the time; "black" resulted in "white" about 60 percent of the time; "man" brought forth "woman" two-thirds of the time; and "good" led to "evil" 80 percent of the time. Even when there is no dominant response, answers typically cluster around related meanings. About 50 percent of the responses to "chair" related in some way to "sitting" and 15 percent related to "table." No one response to "sex" drew more than 10 percent of the answers, but about 40 percent of the total related to gender.

Only the most creative or unsettled individuals step outside the norm. To the word "chair," for which "table" is the single largest response, a creative person might respond "person"; a paranoid might say "electric." Usually, the way to elicit creative responses is to specifically ask for an unusual response rather than the first word that comes to mind.

The word association test was a tool that clinicians used until the 1950s to evaluate a person's mental health. Even today, such tests provide a quick way to gauge the degree to which a person thinks outside the box. Therapists look for atypical responses that might reveal an area of personal distress, such as when the response to "sex" is "sad." Though word association tests are no longer used as a primary diagnostic tool—they now live mostly in the realm of marketing gimmicks and games—they provide insight into how more sophisticated tests can achieve reasonably accurate psychological profiles or provide guidance into potential problem areas. Consider these reactions to the following set of words: me = ugh; you = pain; water = drown; dog = shame; man = man-eater; down = hell. These are actual responses—though not from a single individual. If this pattern of troubled responses *did come* from one person across a battery of associations, we would not have to be trained clinicians to see the potential for a serious psychological problem.

It is not only the response itself that is meaningful, but also the speed of the response. In developing word association tests as a young practitioner, Carl Jung recognized that certain trigger words caused not only an unusual response but also a delay in response—apparently as people unconsciously struggled with an answer to words that had an emotional impact on them. Jung posited that a set of words that caused a delayed response were likely tied to a common underlying emotional issue. His use of the word "complex" to describe these word clusters gave birth to the idiom that someone "has a complex" when struggling with a mental or emotional issue. Because people seemed unaware of delays in their responses, Jung's work provided support for Freud's theory of the unconscious and of repression.

Intrigued at how cognitive preoccupation affects the mind, I developed two word association studies (in print here for the first time). In one study, I distributed a list of ten trigger words and asked for three different responses to each. Then I passed around envelopes containing the ten words. Students drew one of them from the envelope and studied it for thirty seconds. I repeated the original test, asking students to repeat their original responses. Compared to the other words, students were much less likely to repeat their original responses to the word they had studied. Just thirty seconds of stimulus introduced changes in their associations to that word! The effect was so powerful that I could often guess what word they had pulled from the envelope by determining which of their responses had changed the most between the first and second tests.

The other study was similar, requiring three responses each to ten trigger words. Among the trigger words were "hand," "heavy," and "pain." In between the first and second tests, students were asked to hold their hand in the air for four minutes. By the end of that time, they could hardly think of anything but their upraised hand. In the follow-up, the students were far less likely to recall their original responses to the word "hand" than they were the

ASSOCIATIONS THAT ARE NOT ROUTINE

B ecause most word associations are routine, and because the focus of this book is to avoid the routine, two variations on the word association game are worth presenting. The first is "find the middle." We know A and C; what is B? B must be the last half of the word A and the first half of the word C.

A	B	C
Rocking		Person
Hold		Forward
Wall		Wise
Financial		Test

Figure 5–1. Because the first and last words are connected through the word in the middle, the mind cannot default to a routine association. We have to think! Compared to a typical word association game, this one is cognitively stimulating. The answers are, in order: chair, fast, street, and crash. The following "star" game requires similar creativity in finding the source word that links multiple words.

other words on the list. Even if we do nothing more than mention a word to someone and ask them to remember it, they are less likely to recall the word's original associations than if we mention it but do *not* ask them to remember it.

Most of the associations we make between words are stereotypes because we don't think about them. As Jung and others have shown, they do not become significant unless they preoccupy us. *The more we think about a topic, the more our word associations change.* One hospital study that I did was able to determine how fearful patients were by how much their word associations changed while they were waiting for surgery. If "doctor" leads to the response "nurse" on repeated associations, then the patient is not thinking much about the procedure. If "doctor = nurse" becomes "doctor = operation" becomes "doctor = knife," then the patient is continually thinking about the upcoming event, and probably not in a good way.

All of these examples are proof that the unconscious is continually processing information, which is the main point of this section.

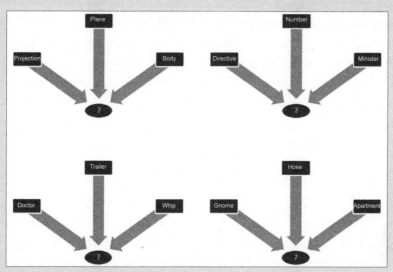

Figure 5-2. What core word links the other three words in each of these puzzles? Typical word association games lead to stereotypical responses; e.g., the word "black" often leads to the answer "white." Little or no thought is required. Games that stymie our default response help stimulate the brain. The "star" association game forces us to search our mind for the original word, resulting in more cognitive effort. (Answers are in the text.)

The second mentally stimulating word association game is the "star," in which three or more words relate to a central word. We know B_1, B_2, and B_3; what is A? The word A must introduce the other words. See Figure 5-2. The answers are, clockwise from top left: astral, prime, garden, and horse.

For an even more exacting game, increase the number of words that relate to the central word without relating to one another. Half the fun is developing these puzzles; the other half is solving the ones our friends create. All kinds of mind games can evolve from this basic idea of finding the hidden connection between seemingly unrelated words or concepts. It's the cognitive version of six degrees of separation.

Most of the time, this is positive, because—as discussed before—unconscious processing is often what creates the unexpected connections that we call creativity. If the brain perceives a stimulus as being threatening, however, as in the surgical example, the shifting associations are evidence of worry. When the threat becomes overwhelming, we cease to think at all, as shown in one final example. While preparing for a major exam, a few students became so stressed that they lost the ability to make any new associations. Whatever the trigger word—"horse," "apple," "couch," etc.—the response was "big." This is the kind of perseveration or stereotype typical of schizophrenics! Under stress, the students developed acute mental rigidity.

DEVELOPING A MECHANIZED STATE OF MIND

Psychologist Abraham Luchins demonstrated how experience quickly causes humans to develop a mechanized state of mind (*einstellung* in German). Luchins set up a series of tests in which subjects had to add or subtract water from three differently sized jars in order to end up with a certain amount of water in any combination of the vessels. Subjects could use only the jars themselves to measure the water volumes.

In the first test, jar A was large enough to hold 21 units of water; jar B, 127 units; jar C, 3 units. The task was to end up with 100 units. The solution was to fill jar B (127), empty it into A (leaving 106 in B); then empty jar B into C (leaving 103); empty C; then empty B into C again. Voilà, 100 units in jar B. Successive tests used different amounts of water in the jars and solved for different amounts, but they all had the same underlying solution: "B minus A minus 2 of C."

The last test involved jars holding 15 units, 39 units, and 3 units, and the task was to measure 18 units. Most subjects solved the problem using the established formula, which they had figured out explicitly or implicitly. Few of them saw the direct solution of filling both A and C (15 + 3 = 18). A control group, which had not been subjected to the series of tests with the more elaborate solution, invariably saw the simpler answer. Luchins also provided yet more proof that stress dramatically increases mental rigidity. In an untimed water-jar test, subjects showed rigidity of thought 70 percent of the time. With time-induced stress, subjects showed rigidity *98 percent* of the time.

A similar form of mental rigidity is seen in what is known as "functional fixedness," which is a pronounced tendency to use an object only for its original purpose even if other uses are beneficial. Karl Duncker gave test subjects a candle, a book of matches, and a box full of thumbtacks. The object was to attach the candle to the wall. Most subjects tried to melt the candle onto the wall or pin it directly via the tacks. Few of the subjects thought to convert the thumbtacks box into a candleholder, attaching the box to the wall with the tacks and placing the candle inside it. Having seen the tacks inside the box, participants could not perceive a novel use for the box. In a later test, subjects were given the same items but the tacks were *not* inside of the box. These participants were twice as likely to solve the problem as those who first saw the box used as a tack container.

Norman Maier asked subjects to tie together two cords hanging from the ceiling, but the cords were just far enough apart that one person could not span the gap. Participants were given various tools, including a pair of pliers, to help solve the problem. Few subjects divined the solution, which was to use the pliers as a weight to swing one cord over to the other. (When subjects were stumped, Maier would casually swing the cord back and forth without otherwise calling attention to his actions. A number of people then solved the problem, unaware that they were keying into the researcher's behavior. Their response to his "priming" is another example of the unconscious at work.)

A variation of the study conducted by Herbert G. Birch and Herbert S. Rabinowitz showed that mental rigidity could still strike the test subjects even if they correctly solved the challenge. First, two groups of subjects did a series of tasks involving the repeated use, respectively, of electrical switches and electrical relays. Both groups were then presented with the two-cord test. The tools provided were switches and relays. Those who had worked with switches tended to use switches as the weight; those who had worked with relays tended to use relays. A control group, which had not been given any tasks before the two-cord experiment, showed no preference for one device over the other.

Rigidity substantially increases with age—more than doubling between the ages of 37 and 61. Generally, children's problem-solving skills improve with age. However, younger children are more capable of seeing new uses for objects than older children or adults. In a test by Margaret Defeyter and Tim German similar to the candle task, children were asked to use a variety of different objects, including a box, to build steps to retrieve an object from a shelf. If the box was not being used as a container when they first saw it, seven-year-olds turned it into a step faster than five-year-olds did. However, if it *was* being used as a container, the five-year-olds did a better job of converting it to a step. Any intended use of the item was equally valid to the younger children. They did not have enough experience with objects to be constrained by conventional wisdom. But symptoms of mental rigidity had already emerged in their elders.

All of these experiments, which illustrate the speed with which we are undone by previous exposure to similar situations, underscore the insidious nature of experience. Rigidity is the extreme form of learning from experience! It not only presents us with very real dangers—as with the Yom Kippur War—but it also curbs the creativity of our thinking.

WHEN IS A HAMMER NOT A HAMMER?

Most of us relapse to old connections even when we think we are doing something new. This unconscious reversion causes us to resist novel experiences, change of any sort. That we think we want change, yet resist it, is especially evident in politics. Slogans such as "time for a change" or the redundant "time for a new beginning" are very effective at winning elections, because all of us can find fault with some aspect of the status quo. But to succeed in getting votes, the call for change needs to be entirely abstract. When any politician (of whatever political stripe) attempts actual change, with a specific agenda in place, opponents very quickly rally their troops about the unknowns or potential downsides of the action. Opposition mounts quickly. In reality our relationship to change is ambivalent. Even if our rational side says we need to pursue new directions, psychologically we prefer the devil we know to the devil we do not.

Our habits are reinforced just enough to cause us to beware of novelty.

Equating similar items is how we make sense of the world, how we learn, how we build civilization. Relying on existing connections (experience) is sufficient for most workaday matters. The really important issues, however—whether personal, business, or political—are too complex and too subtle for us to rely on "close is good enough." These issues are very often similar on the surface but have complicated details and nuances that make them substantially different underneath. Satisficing errors can lead to disastrous decisions and actions in the situations that mean the most to us or have the greatest impact on the world at large. Because weather changes daily and climate by definition changes in terms of decades, it is easy for the average person to experience a month of unseasonably cool weather and dismiss concerns about long-term global warming. A weeklong or monthlong disparity, however, does not offset long-term trends. If the scientists are wrong, their conclusions should be rejected as the result of calm, intensive study and reflection, not as the result of TV sound bites that cater to our predisposition for the status quo.

The studies in this chapter illustrate the folk wisdom that, if we have only a hammer, every problem looks like a nail. Entrenched familiarity causes us to try to fit each new situation into whatever solution we already have in our mental toolkit. We lose the ability to examine our toolkit for new uses. Or to create entirely new tools. The unhindered, if often incoherent, thinking of schizophrenics—not to mention poets and comedians—points the way to the prevention of such mental rigidity. All learning comes from making new connections, not relying on old ones. We must strive to overcome our tendency to settle comfortably into the status quo, both for the sake of the world and for our own mental abilities. We need to invest in doing new things and trying new approaches to even the most routine problems in our lives—*especially* if we think they are unnecessary—to keep our mental systems open and functioning, and to preserve our brainpower.

One way to free ourselves from cognitive rigidity is to step back and abstract the general from the particular. Not only will stepping back stop us from fixating on a particular solution, but it will also open up new possibilities. Whoever said that a hammer is a single-purpose tool? It is a general-purpose tool that, among other things, can act as a weight, door stop, pry-bar, tennis racquet, gavel, sign holder, grappling hook, garden spade, ballast for a toy boat, sounding device to measure fluid levels in a tank, and as a totem and symbol of tribal leadership (see *The Earth Abides*). Sometimes it can even pound nails.

The innovative use of tools brings to mind a trip to Africa, one of my favorite vacation destinations. There are no spare parts in the bush, and the creativity of African auto mechanics is beautiful to watch. Whenever a mechanic sees a bolt or piece of scrap metal, he collects it for future use. All of the garages have boxes of odd metal parts, which all eventually get used. Once, the seat broke on an old Land Rover. The only way to repair it was with an oversized solder-ing iron powered by a propane tank. The flame was so hot that it would have set the cloth seat on fire and burned up the vehicle. After carefully considering the problem, the mechanic left the shop for ten or fifteen minutes. He returned with a bucket of mud and he spread the mud over the seat close to where he needed to work. He added water to keep the mud moist as he made the solder. When he was done, he cleaned the seat and we were on our way. (African ingenuity is unique enough that a website exists to celebrate it: www.Afrigadget.com.)

Compare this incident with the typical experience in the "civi-lized" world. The garage would have ordered a new seat. It would have taken several days to arrive, and the whole fiasco would have cost a fortune. This story is all too familiar to anyone who owns a vehicle. For most problems, the modern mechanic will hook up a diagnostic tool, detect the trouble area, and replace it. No one actu-ally repairs anything anymore. (How many times have we heard a repairperson sagely opine, "The motherboard is shot—need to order a new one"?) All of the things that make life easier also make us less creative. We generally accept the trade-off because modern devices are more reliable and more energy efficient than earlier tech-nology. No one would want to routinely drive a busy highway with a vehicle lacking modern safety systems and designs. The point is twofold: We should get the most out of our technology without letting it enslave us, and we should do hard things on purpose from time to time to stimulate our minds.

Another way to avoid mental inflexibility is to deconstruct a problem rather than trying to tackle it head-on. Software developers examining ways to reuse code are much more likely to succeed if they pull out individual sections and analyze how the separate parts might be used rather than if they try to revise the entire module. By breaking the problem into separate pieces, they untangle their minds from the current utilization.

In general, the best way to confront any problem is to consciously strip away all of our preconceived constraints. A study on matchstick arithmetic found that this strategy was the most effective (yet mentally taxing) way of finding radically different solutions. Matchstick math involves solving problems with sticks that form Roman numerals. We correct an equation by moving one stick. The solution to "IV = III + III" is to move the stick from in front of the "V" to after it, yielding: "VI = III + III." A more difficult problem is to correct this equation: "IX = VI − III." The solution, "IX − VI = III," comes from moving a horizontal "stick" in the operator, thereby flipping the positions of the minus sign and the equal sign. Treating an operator as a stick is permissible, but because the trick is not called out in advance, most people overlook it as a possibility. When moving one of the sticks in the numerals—the *einstellung* approach—does not work, people are forced to consider new options. Eventually, most people figure out the answer. The solutions to most riddles come from relaxing our mental constraints about the question. The same can be applied to all questions. We do not have to wait until we are actually blocked. We can discipline ourselves to try new approaches to every significant problem we face.

Escaping the status quo requires intention—whether it is for simple wordplay, for math puzzles, or for real situations, decisions, and actions. When Luchins said "Don't be blind!" to his water-test subjects, more than half of them broke out of their mental inflexibility and were able to see the simpler solution. Later, he found that having students write "Don't be blind!" as they began tests helped them avoid falling into mental rigidity. Just being aware of our tendency to fall into mental inflexibility helps us avoid it.

Simple changes can also help us overcome our innate mental inflexibility, as shown by what happens when we travel to a new city. After just a few hours, we begin to develop a cognitive map of the area. We figure out that we turn left at the corner to get to the coffee shop and right to see the cathedral. We find landmarks that guide us back to our hotel. Mastering an unfamiliar environment is perceived as pleasurable. New connections occur. New circuits form. Without trying, we begin to maximize our brainpower. The antidote to the boredom and waste of routine existence—and the rigidity and decline that sets in so early in life—is to put ourselves in situations in which we are not masters! Temporary mental discomfort is the trade-off for challenging the brain, pulling it out of its habitual mode, and stimulating new connections and capabilities. Like climbing a mountain, we can achieve mental success—and mental pleasure—only when we expend energy.

===== LESSONS IN BRAINPOWER =====

- Behaviors learned by partial and inconsistent reinforcement resist change and are exceedingly difficult to extinguish. Because very few circumstances in the world provide consistent feedback, old habits continue even when there is *more support* for new ways of doing things.
- Our basic conservatism as a species comes from *satisfycing,* a psychological term that means we stop searching when we find a solution that is good enough.
- The brain will often make the easiest connections—those based on experience—rather than the best connections—those based on new information.
- Many psychological tests show that rigidity of thought develops rapidly with even small amounts of experience. Rigidity increases substantially with age, illustrating the cumulative impact of our reliance on experience.
- In order to break mental habits, we must consciously strip away all of our preconceived constraints. Being aware of our tendency to fall into mental inflexibility helps us avoid it.

PART II

THE CASE FOR HEAVY MENTAL LIFTING

HOW THE CHALLENGES WE GIVE OUR BRAINS AFFECT OUR HEALTH, LONGEVITY, AND INTELLIGENCE

SIX

The Font of Cognitive Fitness

Mike and Jim are close friends, school and neighborhood buddies. Raised in the same environment, they enjoy similar activities and share many of the same friends. They marry at about the same time and spend their adult lives in the same town. As they reach their golden years, however, Mike has *three times* the likelihood of developing Alzheimer's disease as his friend.

What accounts for this startling difference?

Jim went to college. Mike didn't.

People who have gone to college have *one-third* the likelihood of developing Alzheimer's or another frightening, degenerative brain disease compared to everyone else. People who have a higher education decrease their risk of dementia by two-thirds!

Scientists from Britain and Finland have discovered that every year of higher education results in an 11 percent decrease in the risk of developing dementia. *Four years of college and two years of graduate school will reduce the risk by 66 percent.* Though this report is the most dramatic, many other studies also demonstrate the substantial benefits of education. Eight separate cohorts (groups of people who are statistically similar) from France, Sweden, Finland, China, and the United States, indicate a correlation between higher education and cognitive vitality later in life. A pooled analysis of four other European studies, plus separate research in New York City, shows a tie between literacy and cognitive ability in older adults. Literacy does not necessarily prevent the biological decline associated with dementia, but it may compensate for it and thus postpone the onset of symptoms—hopefully beyond our lifetime. (More about this important distinction in the next chapter.)

A cautious reader must first ask this question: Does our environment improve our cognitive abilities, or do people with superior cognitive abilities—including resistance to dementia—simply outperform everyone else? Are we born cognitively great, or do we become cognitively great through education and other life experiences? Let us begin, then, by examining how childhood intelligence unfolds and how this unfolding relates to education and other aspects of the environment.

NATURE VERSUS NURTURE: HOW MUCH ADVANTAGE IS BUILT IN?

The impact of "nature versus nurture" on our intelligence has been argued since Darwin's day with all kinds of social as well as scientific ramifications. If genes determine our success in life, then poverty proves the inferiority of the poor, and there's nothing to be done about it. This argument was for generations the last major prop of the British aristocracy. The "divine right of kings" morphed into the "divine right of genes," as illustrated by the aristocracy's superior bank accounts and their control of the political system, which conveniently maintained their economic advantages. Similar arguments are raised today about the value of spending tax dollars on the poor, who generally have low IQ scores. If their personal outcomes are largely predetermined by their genes, why bother? And, in truth, most researchers believed until recently that our cognitive abilities were relatively fixed, if not at birth, then at least after the explosive cognitive growth of early childhood.

Psychologist Arthur Jenson, the epitome of the "gene" side, has been arguing with impressive statistical support since 1969 that intelligence is largely heritable. (He has also raised controversy by claiming race-based differences in intelligence, that Asians are superior to whites and whites are superior to blacks in abstract reasoning.) When asked the extent to which environmental factors can boost innate intelligence, he replied, "Not much." A number of studies, in addition to Jensen's, seem to prove the superiority of genes in determining intelligence. Studies of twins who are raised separately, for instance, show that in adulthood the twins tend to have IQs more akin to their biological parents than to their adoptive parents. The American Psychological Association puts the correlation between heritability and IQ at "around .75" (1.0 indicates a perfect correlation).

Yet other reputable scientists, supported by an equally impressive array of studies, have shown the positive impact of an enriched environment for children. New European immigrant groups to the United States and white Appalachian children scored well below average on intelligence tests in the 1930s, yet later generations were normal. IQ scores have risen substantially worldwide since World War II. For example, IQs in the Netherlands and in Israel have increased twenty points in just one generation. Such dramatic short-term changes are more likely to result from documented improvements in education during those times than from the glacial pace of genetic mutation.

What gives?

One answer is the inherent difficulty of measuring the many aspects of intelligence in a clear and discrete way and then ascribing the results to any one cause. In seeking to make sense of complex data on the heritability of intelligence, most researchers assume that inborn traits are additive. That is, three separate intellectual traits with a benefit of 5 percent each would result in a 15 percent advantage. Yet an individual's traits arise through complex genetic interactions in a manner that is anything but additive. A person whose father is nine inches taller than normal and whose mother is six inches taller than normal will not automatically grow to be fifteen inches taller than normal. The odds are good that he or she will be taller than normal, but the difference might be a little or a lot. The child could even be shorter. Similarly, it is highly unlikely that a number of genetic differences in intelligence will add up to the cumulative, overwhelming advantage that some researchers claim. The environment itself—while a child is in the womb and even during early childhood—also affects how genes are expressed. For example, malnutrition in a pregnant woman can result in an increased risk of diabetes and heart disease for her child and excessive stress hormones in a pregnant woman can result in greater watchfulness and reactivity in her child. Similarly, severe stress in early childhood alters DNA expression in a way that can lead to speech, behavior, and mental problems.

ENVIRONMENT MATTERS

Psychologist Eric Turkheimer sheds some light on the interplay of nature and nurture. Recognizing that all of the twin studies showing the heritability of IQ had been done with middle-class or wealthy families, Turkheimer repeated the studies with 320 pairs of twins from exceedingly poor families. For them, he found that genetics played a *tiny role* in the development of intelligence. If 1.0 is a 100 percent correlation between genes and brains, the ratio in wealthy families was 0.72, but the ratio in poor families was only 0.10. Turkheimer found that the environment played *four times* the role in the outcome of intelligence for poor families compared to wealthy families.

From this standpoint, a positive environment does not play an enabling role so much as a negative environment plays a disabling role—at least in childhood. In one respect, this is common sense. If we plant two genetically identical seeds of corn, one in well-nourished soil and the other in poor soil, it is not surprising when the seed in the good soil grows twice as tall. The same is true for the cognitive abilities of human beings in our own cultural gardens. If we all have a sufficiently stimulating environment, then our inherent abilities—our genetic gifts—will dominate in the unfolding of our lives. If we lack a sufficiently stimulating environment, our cognitive gifts never have the chance to blossom. The most extreme example of the latter exists in the form of severely neglected children (often in overwhelmed orphanages in poor countries) who are left in their beds almost nonstop, sometimes never fully developing.

A nurturing environment can also multiply otherwise modest genetic advantages, as W. T. Dickens and J. R. Flynn describe in their complex and artful analysis titled "The IQ Paradox Resolved." Their math is daunting, but their central example is beguilingly simple. A child has inborn basketball skills that are 10 percent above average. He plays regularly in the backyard with his bigger and stronger brothers, improving his skills enough that he joins the more advanced players on the playground. Motivated by his enjoyment and success, he cajoles his parents into sending him to summer basketball camp, where he draws the attention of a coach who encourages him to try out for the school team. He plays for four years against the best players in the state. Eventually, he goes on to play college ball.

When he started, the skill level of this youth was at the 60th percentile—10 percent better than the norm. When he completes his career, he is at the 95th percentile. His steady improvement over the years appears to have been driven by the unfolding of his genetic abilities—coordination, strength, speed. In actuality, his success *began* with his genetic endowments, which propelled him into continually more challenging and enriching environments, which pushed his skills further. His environment helped him turn his minor genetic advantage into a major one. Standard studies have not accounted for this cycle of positive reinforcement between inherited abilities and the external world. The environmental side of skill development is masked.

Similar "gene times environment" pressure occurs with most children from the middle and upper classes who are endowed with even small cognitive advantages. Their skill at reading or math or music draws the support of parents, who treat them with more books, laptops, and musical instruments. These children are encouraged by their teachers to take more challenging courses or enter talented and gifted programs. All along, they interact with other smart kids. They might even spend their summers at math or music camp. Increasing this multiplier is the fact that the best teachers often end up at desirable schools, where their interaction with high-performing students and other good teachers tends to raise school performance even more. The lack of such social multipliers among most disadvantaged children—in academics as opposed to athletics—helps explain much of the disparity in their IQ scores and scholarly performance. This is no surprise to teachers, who lament unsupportive parents and the lack of cognitive stimuli or focus in many less-advantaged homes. The result is too often children who are not only unprepared but also unmotivated.

From these different sources we can piece together a rational perspective on the development of native intelligence. Our genetic endowments, coupled with many early environmental impacts, establish our childhood intelligence. An environment lacking a sufficient level of stimulation stifles our mental development. An environment with a sufficient level of stimulation enables our genetically different abilities to flower, and at the same time often sets into motion positive social and cultural pressures that reinforce our improvement. All of these factors unite to establish our childhood intelligence, which becomes the baseline of our cognitive vitality in adulthood.

INTELLIGENCE, IQ, AND COGNITION

Before moving forward, we should discuss the difference between intelligence, IQ, and cognition. The common characterization of intelligence is the capacity to learn and understand, to solve problems, and to reason abstractly. However, there are as many different formal definitions as there are theorists, and every definition is in some way lacking. Few theories account for creativity or for emotional intelligence, which is the ability to work constructively with other people. Whatever its definition, intelligence is best conceived as the sum of all our different mental abilities and how successfully we apply them in the real world. Reaching our full potential for these diverse mental abilities is what we mean by "maximizing brainpower."

IQ (the "intelligence quotient") is a number that measures a subset of our intelligence on the basis of standardized tests. IQ tests are useful because high and low scores reasonably predict academic and professional success and identify students with special needs. IQ tests have been faulted for focusing primarily on "book learning," for treating intelligence as if it were one dimensional—and reducible to a single number—and for being culturally biased. An immigrant to a new culture or a minority who operates outside of common cultural and language norms will usually fare worse on these tests. Cultural bias can be minimized but never eliminated. A person's IQ number can also rise or fall over time. It does not have a static meaning. The concept is dynamic: What is our IQ on a certain date and under certain circumstances?

Perhaps "IQ" should instead be called something like the "achievement predictor" because the research shows that someone who does well on an IQ test has greater chances of achieving success than someone who does poorly. These predictions are not equal, however, to native intelligence. A low score on an IQ test may indicate any number of things—from low intelligence to special needs, serious ignorance, or a type of intelligence that the test cannot measure—artistic ability, for instance. The IQ test has few false positives but many potentially false negatives.

Cognition means something altogether different. Generally, cognition is considered to be the "process of thought," the way in which the brain processes information. Of the many aspects of cognition, the most important are attention, perception, and short-term memory. These are the brain's primary tasks when it faces new information. We must attend to new data or it never registers; it is simply lost. Once the stimulus is registered, we must then perceive the data; for example, the brain must translate light patterns into a meaningful image, and sound waves into words or music. We must hold the information in our memory bank until the brain decides whether it is important enough to retain. If it is not, we delete it. The amount of information we can fit into interim storage is important because it affects how much information we can process at any one time. Providing the basic tools of information processing, cognition is the gatekeeper to all of the brain's other marvelous functions.

Because new information is constantly flowing in, pushing out previous information, it is difficult to keep data in temporary storage for any duration. Speed of cognition is thus very important. Slow processing has the same effect as reduced storage. Most people's auditory neurons, for example, require about thirty milliseconds after hearing one sound before they are ready to process the next. Eighty percent of children with delays in language development, however, require at least three times as long. Is it a surprise that these kids have language and speech difficulties, when they are processing (as opposed to physically hearing) only one out of every three or four sounds? It would be like trying to learn language over a spotty cellphone connection. (Scientists are working on ways to help bring the internal processing of these kids up to normal.)

In general, the speed of cognitive processing declines with age. The level of the decline varies from person to person, but the drop is universal. Thankfully, the decline is usually not severe enough to seriously disrupt our day-to-day lives. My cognitive skills, for instance, have declined enough that I should not be flying fighter planes. Fortunately, that requirement does not come up often in my line of work. I do, however, retain the cognitive speed to drive automobiles. The same is true for most septuagenarians and octogenarians. Plaguing Florida and other areas with large senior populations, poor-performing elderly drivers have trouble with vision and hearing or suffer from other physical ills (including the side effects of some medications). As frightening as they can be, most of these drivers do not have a problem with cognition per se.

All IQ tests require the use of basic cognition. When we take IQ tests, we have to attend, perceive, and process information, and we have to do it in a reasonable amount of time. In fact, everything we do requires attention, perception, and short-term memory, including what the reader is doing now to make sense of the words on this page. For our purposes, IQ, though important, is just one metric of intelligence. Having been broadly used for more than a hundred years, IQ numbers can help us compare general intellectual or educational levels from generation to generation and from group to group or society to society. It can be useful as long as we treat IQ as an approximation for general cognitive skills, but not as the definition, or epitome, of intelligence.

THE MANY PATHS TO PROTECTING THE BRAIN

Much of our cognitive ability as adults relates directly to our childhood intelligence, which has a strong genetic component, but a good deal also comes from our experiences afterward. Much of what happens after childhood depends on education and what happens as the result of education.

The work of K. Warner Schaie stands out as a major contribution to the research about cognition, and what aspects of life affect it the most. Schaie has spent most of his professional life carrying out the Seattle Longitudinal Study and analyzing data from it. A longitudinal study is one that follows a population group over the course of many years, in contrast to the usual cross-sectional study of different age groups done at one time. Cross-sectional studies are flawed because they may show differences that appear to be age related when, in fact, they are cohort related. If we reviewed the Netherland's IQ test scores on a cross-sectional basis, for example, we might conclude that IQ declines twenty points as we age because the IQ of the average sixty-year-old person was twenty points lower than that of the average forty-year-old person. A longitudinal approach would show instead that the IQ of the older generation was *always* lower than that of the younger. The IQ of Mr. Jones Sr. did not decline with age; rather, the IQ of Mr. Jones Jr. was higher than his father's, most likely because of improved schooling. If the IQ of the elder cohort had, in fact, declined, a longitudinal study would show that, too.

Having access to a Seattle health maintenance organization (HMO), Schaie took a random sample of between about 600 and 900 people of various age groups from the large pool of subscribers. He and his colleagues did six cycles of studies, one every seven years, replenishing the groups with representative replacements to account for attrition. Because the HMO provided health insurance, which many poor people in the United States do not have, the cohorts were slightly skewed toward the higher end of the socioeconomic spectrum. With the support of the HMO, researchers were able to track the subjects' health as well as their cognitive vitality.

Because of the number of population groups studied and the number of years of follow-up testing, Schaie could follow cognitive trends as people aged. He could also look back to determine the cause of these trends. He asked: Which people are doing much better cognitively than the others, and what did they do in their lives to account for the difference? His ability to answer this question underlines the importance of following the same people over time rather than taking snapshots of a population at a single point in time. The cognitive abilities of some people declined rapidly with age, while other people remained very sharp mentally despite age. Schaie uncovered a stark rule: *People who challenged their brains throughout life did better than those who did not.*

In his many reports over the decades of the study, Schaie found overall that there was little or no cognitive decline by age sixty and consistent but not severe decline by age seventy-four. Even so, at age eighty-one, more than half of the subjects showed no decline over the previous seven years. Some octogenarians did as well as adolescents on verbal tests. Most important, decline was highly variable rather than uniform. People declined or maintained on an individual basis.

The ability of people to maintain their cognitive fitness was linked to a number of factors: high level of education; high socioeconomic status; complex and intellectually stimulating work; good friendships and social interactions; the high cognitive status of a spouse; and a flexible personal lifestyle, particularly from middle age on.

Among all the groups in the study, the people who did the best had a high socioeconomic status and a high degree of interaction with their work and life. The next best at maintaining cognitive fitness were people of average socioeconomic status who also had a high degree of involvement in life. At the bottom end were the people with the lowest education and income, and the most disengagement from life. In many cases, these were widowed homemakers. Cognitive decline was also related to family dissolution and cardiovascular or other chronic disease.

No researcher believes that education in and of itself provides protection against dementia. A professor for many decades, I can attest that college does not provide a sophistication of thought or a well of deep wisdom that can protect us from brain disease for decades to come. Additional years of study, particularly if they involve a variety of subjects, will undoubtedly lift a person's cognitive capacity. What is more important, though, is that a good education opens a number of paths to cognitive fitness. In addition to the greater professional and economic status and the accompanying enriched social milieu, related benefits for the highly educated include improved health and lifestyle choices, a safer work environment, and a better grip on ways to handle stress. Most critically, people who have college educations generally have more interesting and demanding jobs than those who do not. In many ways, a person's level of education is an easy-to-determine indicator of the challenges that his or her brain is likely to face during his or her professional life. This is borne out in Schaie's work, in which education is the linchpin for all of the factors that play a role in maintaining cognitive fitness. Other studies show that higher education, a demanding occupation, and devotion to leisure activities, all have separate, synergistic effects on a person's cognitive fitness.

Researchers have looked at the overall complexity of occupations along with the nature of the work—whether the occupation primarily involves people (sales, human resources, etc.), things (construction, manufacturing, etc.), or data (financial analysis, software programming, etc.). The results are mostly, but not completely, consistent. Let's take a look.

A "Complexity of Work" study from the Canadian Study of Health and Aging, involving 3,557 subjects over ten years, concluded that a high complexity of work reduced the risk of dementia by an average of 27 percent for jobs involving things and 34 percent for jobs involving people. The research also showed that it was important how *much* of a person's career was spent working in complex jobs as the primary occupation. If the length of time was less than the median time of the group as a whole (twenty-three years in this study), the complex job lowered the risk of dementia but not of Alzheimer's. If the length of time was more than the median time of the group, the complex occupation protected against Alzheimer's, too.

The degree of protection offered by long-term complex work is staggering. For long-term jobs involving things, the risk was reduced *55 percent* for dementia and *52 percent* for Alzheimer's. For long-term jobs involving people, the risk was reduced *64 percent* for dementia and *69 percent* for Alzheimer's. Here is yet more confirmation that cognitively stimulating activities reduce the risk of dementia by two-thirds.

Jobs involving complexity with data had mixed results. In the Canadian study, shorter-term complex occupations involving data generally had no impact on cognitive health, but longer-term jobs actually *increased* the risk of dementia and Alzheimer's. Researchers speculated that data-related jobs might have been more stressful or more socially isolating, offsetting the benefits of complexity. Negative results were limited to men, possibly because women tend to have stronger social networks both inside and outside of work.

Two studies from Sweden, however, showed that occupational complexity involving data (as well as people) had a significant benefit to cognitive health. One showed complexity with data led to higher performance on verbal, spatial, and mental speed of calculation. The other showed that people whose occupations involved complexity with people and data scored consistently higher on cognitive tests than those whose occupations were less mentally demanding. The impact of occupation was separate from any impact caused by age, sex, childhood circumstances, or education.

The converse of these findings also applies. The earlier people retire, the faster their memories decline. The cause is unclear but it is likely a combination of reduced mental effort, reduced social engagement, and a relatively inactive retirement.

In general, jobs involving substantial physical activity lead to an increased risk of dementia and Alzheimer's, presumably because such jobs offer less cognitive stimulation. Another possibility is that the increased risk of injuries (including head injuries) might lead to reduced activity over time and less overall stimulation in life.

LEISURE ACTIVITIES AND SOCIAL NETWORKS

Let's take a look at some other activities that offer cognitive protection. New York City studies showed that reading, board games, music, and dancing all fall into this category and, in general, high leisure activity reduced the risk of dementia by 38 percent. A Cleveland study showed that people who kept their minds active in midlife were three times less likely to develop Alzheimer's than people who did not. A Swedish study showed that cognitively healthy older women were marked by active daily lives, strong social networks, and healthy physical behaviors. A French study showed that such diverse activities as traveling, odd jobs, and knitting all lowered the risk of dementia. Leisure pursuits that are mentally effortful help protect us from Alzheimer's independently from other factors, but almost *any* leisure activity helps reduce the risk of dementia.

Exercise, too, has serious benefits for the brain. Dozens of studies show a reduced chance of dementia or Alzheimer's for those who exercise the most. We can predict a person's future cognitive fitness based on how much he or she exercises today. In follow-ups ranging from five to seven years after the original studies, regular exercisers were found to reduce their risk of dementia between 20 and 50 percent. A study of 1,740 people in Seattle showed that people over the age of sixty-five who exercised three times or more a week had a 38 percent lower risk of serious mental decline.

Aerobic training provides the most direct benefit, though a combination of weight training and aerobic training may improve brain function more than aerobic work alone. Women seem to get particular benefit from exercise, and—in older women—exercise seems to offset the possible negative side effects of long-term hormone replacement therapy. Though most studies focus on older people, research has discovered positive correlations between exercise and cognitive vitality in people of all ages. Several studies also indicate that exercise, particularly out of doors, helps improve concentration for people with attention deficit hyperactivity disorder (ADHD).

We need not despair if we are not athletic champions, setting age-group records in weightlifting or the 800-meter run. The benefit of exercise is greatest for those who are currently the least physically active. This makes sense if we remember that change is the brain's best friend. Let's say that we live in Honolulu and walk two miles a day. If we walk another half a mile, we will not dramatically increase the blood flow to our brains or increase our cognitive stimulation. Now let's say we're watching television in Honolulu. A news bulletin informs us that people from the island who walk two or more miles a day reduce their chance of developing dementia by

40 percent compared to coach potatoes like us. We set down our snack, strap on our walking shoes, and head for the beach. On this walk, we stimulate the balance, coordination, and navigation centers in our brain. We kindle the visual, auditory, and olfactory centers with new sights, sounds, and smells. Our skin feels new sensations from the breeze and the sun's warmth, and reports them to our brain. We observe the personal interactions among families and probably note a budding romance or two, which, in turn, rouses old memories about our own youthful romps on the beach. We might pet a dog or return an errant Frisbee. We will likely visit, however briefly, with some of the people we meet. And of course we significantly raise the blood flow to our brain compared to our sedentary activities. Even if we walk just half a mile this first time, a host of new stimuli will flood the brain. The result is a greater cognitive surge than if we were already out and had merely increased our distance.

A *variety* of exercise is a stronger predictor of cognitive health than the *total amount* of exercise. Again, this makes sense because water aerobics stimulates the brain differently than walking, bicycling, golfing, or playing tennis. (Cross-training is also good for the different muscle groups.) It's more important to participate in an assortment of activities than any one activity, however cognitively challenging. And getting a friend to participate also increases the potential benefit. It ups the odds that we will actually go for that jog or play that round of golf, and the social stimulation also increases our cognitive engagement.

The cognitive engagement that comes from human interactions—especially friendships or other close relationships—creates many of the benefits that come from all leisure activities, including exercise. The importance of a healthy social life may, in fact, explain the contradictory studies related to the impact of alcohol on our health. An excess of alcohol is bad for us, but some studies show that a modest amount of red wine is good for us; others show that a modest amount of white wine is good for us; and still others are inconclusive. We should *not*, however, heed the advice of some pundits who claim that we should drink a glass of wine for our health before we go to bed each night. It is very likely that people who drink modestly do so over a good meal and in the company of good friends. Light alcohol use may be masking the real benefit—pleasant personal interactions with others. In a cognitive comparison of similar groups of seniors from the United States and England, the English had an advantage in only one area: the English who drank moderately performed better on cognitive tests than the Americans, many of whom were abstainers. The likely explanation is that, in England, most of the drinkers in this age group benefitted from the social stimulation of their local pub.

This last comparative study also showed, in rather startling terms, the impact of our occupational and social environment over the course of a lifetime. The comparison of the cognitive health of seniors in England against seniors in the United States showed that the people in the United States did "significantly better" than their cohorts in England—and the advantage increased with age. *The Americans did better—despite being in generally worse physical health.* Of the sample, 16 percent of the Americans had diabetes versus 9 percent of the English; 57 percent had hypertension versus 45 percent; and 18 percent had cancer versus 8 percent. Yet overall performance on cognitive tests gave the Americans a ten-year cognitive advantage over the English. The seventy-five-year-old Americans had the mental fitness of the sixty-five-year-old English.

Given that physical health and vigor tends to promote cognitive fitness, how is it that the unhealthy Americans outperformed the healthy English in cognitive results? The primary factors were higher education and greater wealth, along with lower levels of depression among the U.S. subjects. Though the Americans had greater hypertension, they also took more medication, which offset the negative impact. Depression among the English caused the highest proportion of cognitive decline. The English smoked and drank more, but the drinking was problematic only when it was done in excess.

IT ALL ADDS UP

Our cognitive skills are not fixed. At all ages the brain has the ability to respond to new information and new stimuli. Our intellectual abilities are a combination of our inherent genetic gifts and the lifelong consequences of all of the decisions we make that either positively or negatively contribute to our cognitive fitness. Though childhood ability has the strongest single impact on our cognitive function later in life, the cumulative impacts of education, career, and lifestyle can have effects that are at least as powerful. We probably won't get a 66 percent cognitive improvement from six years of college-level study; another 66 percent increase from a challenging job; a 30 plus percent gain from interesting personal activities; plus another 30 plus percent gain from exercise. As with genetic effects, the numbers are not additive.

However, just about everything we choose to do can direct our cognition up or down. The effect may be negligible or significant, but it all adds up. The more challenging choices we make, and the longer we do them, the greater the benefit—usually by a considerable amount. It does not really matter whether we work primarily with people, things, or data. What matters is whether the work is challenging or routine. Schaie shows that we need to remain engaged. As is implied in his studies and demonstrated in others, a variety of stimulation matters a great deal to our brainpower.

Unlike our genetic predisposition, over which we have little control, we can control the uses to which we put our lives and our brains. Whether the reduced risk for dementia is 30, 50, or even close to 70 percent, there is no other change we can make in our lives that can affect the health of our brain as much as seeking cognitively stimulating practices in everything we do. No genetic variability can account for such a difference. No breakthrough medical treatment or expensive new designer drug will have an impact remotely as large. At least not in our lifetimes. By engaging our brains throughout our lives, by maximizing our brainpower, we protect our minds. Challenging the brain helps maintain cognitive vigor and capacity. And maintaining our cognitive health maintains our quality of life.

What if, however, we did not hit the books as youths? What if our current occupation is not all that stimulating? What if we are older and reflect back on a life that was a good deal less challenging than we now wish it had been? A personal example may be of use here. When I was twelve, a few years after World War II, I made the difficult decision to leave my family behind in central Europe and immigrate to Israel on my own. For five years, I lived and worked on a collective farm. For four years on the kibbutz, I did not read a single book. Eventually, I returned to school, and I have largely lived the life of an academic ever since. It is unlikely that the four-year gap in my education created any long-term harm to my cognition. Not knowing the language of my new country, and becoming a teenager in a new environment without family support, presented a number of challenges that I had to overcome. Reading is not the only way to get information or to challenge the brain.

We cannot change the past. We cannot overcome whatever childhood cognitive deficit we may now carry with us. We can change only the present and the future. We focus on what we can control. We can seek more stimulating work, or more stimulating activities outside of work. If we do not have the money to spend on engaging trips to the Riviera, we can find stimulation enough at local parks, in the woods, or on a public beach. If we did not study in our youth, we can study now. If we find this difficult, all the better! It means the brain is being challenged. We can use public libraries to increase our reading or to learn a new language. We can join book clubs. We can explore the world's knowledge on the Internet. Regardless of age, we can take classes informally or work toward a degree. Many middle-aged and elderly people go back to complete college—or even high school. Someone once wrote an advice columnist wondering if age was an impediment to seeking a medical degree. "I will be forty when I'm done in seven years," the person said. The columnist replied, "How old will you be in seven years if you don't go to medical school?" After a career in the army, an acquaintance returned to school to obtain a degree in counseling. Rather than retire, he now helps other veterans make the transition back to civilian life. The veterans are better for it, and so is he. Perhaps the greatest example is George Dawson, who learned to read at the age of ninety-eight and then wrote his autobiography at the age of one hundred.

In our past, what was not done . . . was not done. It is great if we invested in our cognitive bank account early, but we can still make deposits any time we choose. *The very act of trying will mint new cognitive coin.* A forty-year-old who gains 20 percent—or an eighty-year-old who gains 10 percent!—will knock a few years off his or her cognitive age. If we cannot reset our childhood intelligence, we can certainly roll back the clock.

Sooner is better, but it is never too late.

=== **LESSONS IN BRAINPOWER** ===

- Higher education decreases the risk of dementia *by two-thirds.* It is not that college itself creates deep pools of wisdom but rather that it opens up a world of more interesting and challenging work.
- Full development of our mental abilities usually comes as the result of "gene times environment": Genetic endowments lead us to stimulating environments, which improve our performance and take us to even more stimulating environments in a positive cycle of reinforcement. The opposite is also true. In a non-stimulating environment, our innate abilities may never blossom.
- IQ is best thought of as a predictor of success. High scores predict academic and professional success; low scores predict the opposite. But IQ relates as much to social and economic circumstances as to intelligence.
- The cognitive abilities of some people decline rapidly with age, while other people remain mentally sharp despite age. People who challenge their brains throughout life do better than those who do not.
- We can predict future cognitive fitness based on how people are living their life today. The more complex the work they do, the more leisure activities they participate in, and the more they exercise, the better they will fare cognitively.
- Variety in leisure activities and exercise is more important to cognitive health than the total amount of activities, because each thing we do stimulates the brain in different ways.
- We cannot control our genetic predisposition to dementia, but we can control the amount of effort we demand of our minds. Challenging our brains throughout our lives will do more to protect the health of our brain than any other factor, genetic or medical.

SEVEN

Build Cognitive Reserves

Let's revisit Mike. Though he did not attend college, Mike is a go-getter. He starts his own business and engages in civic affairs. He can't afford long trips, but he camps and fishes and explores every state and national park he can reach by car. He's an avid reader. As a result of all of these adult activities, he reduces his risk for dementia by, let's say, 20 percent.

We now face another question, one that is important to understanding the biology of the brain, the unfolding of dementia, and the ways we can avoid or delay it. Does cognitive stimulation prevent, slow, or halt the progress of brain disease, or does it somehow *offset* the effects of brain disease? Do Mike and all of the cognitively fit people from the last chapter develop fewer physical problems in their brains than typical people of their age? Or are they developing the same disease processes as other people but are better able to withstand them?

To answer this question, we must heed Hamlet's advice and get ourselves to a nunnery. Religious communities are excellent research vehicles in medicine because the similar and stable living conditions control for most of the environmental variables of the people involved. Research on religious orders and lay groups who practice similarly abstemious diets and lifestyles have helped confirm the connection between diet and ailments such as heart disease and cancer. The finding that nuns have lower rates of cervical cancer but higher rates of breast cancer led to an investigation of the impact of celibacy on both diseases. It turns out that while celibacy protects against cervical cancer, because the predominant cause of the disease is a virus transmitted during sex, hormonal changes during pregnancy lower the rate of breast cancer.

We also have learned a tremendous amount about the brain, aging, and dementia as the result of the famous nun studies performed by David Snowdon and his colleagues. (These studies are so well regarded among psychologists that they are invariably prepended with the adjective "famous.")

Snowdon is an epidemiologist and professor of neurology who has studied 678 Catholic nuns in one order for more than twenty-five years. The nuns ranged in age from seventy-five to one hundred and six. Participants agreed to have regular cognitive tests; eventually, most of them also agreed to let their brains be autopsied after their deaths so that scientists could correlate the physical state of their brains with their cognitive history and (for most) their eventual mental decline.

Early on, Snowdon discovered that every nun had written a one-page biographical sketch when she first entered the order, at the average age of twenty-two. He and his team developed an analysis of the cognitive sophistication of the biographies on the basis of "idea density," the number of separate ideas that appeared in each of them. If their biographies were of equal length, a nun with twenty distinct ideas would have twice the idea density of a nun with ten distinct ideas. (Technically, the essays were measured in terms of the number of ideas for every ten words.) Each nun's biography was scored and compared with her current cognitive ability, at the average age of eighty. Thirty-five percent of the nuns who had shown low idea density at age twenty-two showed mental impairment on standard tests at age eighty, compared to only 2 percent of those who had shown high idea density at age twenty-two. Even more strikingly, 90 percent of the nuns who developed Alzheimer's had shown low idea density at age twenty-two versus only 13 percent of the healthy sisters. Snowdon could predict which of the nuns would get Alzheimer's disease sixty years later by evaluating their youthful autobiographies!

This dramatic correlation between the nuns' cognitive power in young adulthood and in old age led Snowdon's team to discount the effect of later influences on cognitive vitality. The researchers themselves had a hard time accepting these results; one found the lack of impact of later education or occupation to be "bizarre."

Yet many of the nuns featured in Snowdon's book *Aging With Grace* benefited from education and stimulating occupations, as described in our last chapter. Ninety percent of the nuns were teachers, and 45 percent had master's degrees or more. Of the nuns who maintained their cognitive gifts well into their senior years, many obtained advanced degrees or adopted leadership roles in schools and other institutions in middle age or later. Most of them continued to work well past the normal age of retirement. They did a lifetime of complex work with both people *and* data.

Sister Dolores, for example, obtained her bachelor's degree at age twenty-nine; her master's degree at forty-four; a second master's in a different field at fifty-one; and a PhD at fifty-five. She led a reforestation effort in Africa at age sixty-seven and learned computers at seventy-six. Her occupational exploits were typical of the nuns who maintained their cognitive vitality throughout their lives. Sister Nicolette, who began teaching school at age sixteen (before she had her own high school diploma), eventually earned her bachelor's and master's degrees, taught in a number of schools, and was still active at age seventy-nine, frequently traversing the hilly streets of her town to visit the sick and homebound. Another nun proudly announced that she had taught college for forty-eight years, missing only two days of work.

Rather than indicating that occupation has little impact on our cognitive health, Snowdon's study may actually prove the opposite. The young women who demonstrated intellectual strengths (as evidenced in their biographies) were encouraged to become teachers or to take career paths that led to leadership roles within schools or the religious organization—the church's "fast track." The less intellectually talented young women generally took less challenging roles within the order, often unskilled ones. The problem may not be that the cognitive differences of youth were set in genetic stone but that the less stimulating work of the lower-performing nuns maintained and reinforced their "low idea density" across six decades. Like the young basketball player who started out with a minor talent, which was cultivated by increasingly challenging environments, the nuns who had the greatest natural gifts took paths that accentuated them.

THE TERRIBLE COST OF COGNITIVE DECLINE

Though most researchers disagree with his conclusion that occupation has no influence on later cognitive vitality, Snowdon's studies are important because they connect cognitive fitness with reasonable conclusiveness to when and how dementia develops.

Dementia is a broad term used to indicate significant mental decline. It is a symptom of an underlying organic cause, usually classed as either vascular or Alzheimer's. Vascular dementia can be caused by several different problems, all of which directly kill brain cells: a hemorrhage that leaks blood into brain tissue; a clot that lodges in a small artery and cuts off blood flow; or a vascular spasm that has the same effect. The cause can also be organic or external in the form of a blow to the head. With vascular dementia, the patient's suffering is proportionate to the severity and location of the damage, which can sometimes be reduced by immediate medical treatment. Smaller strokes often leave us with most, if not all, of our mental faculties intact, though we will likely suffer from loss of speech, loss of movement in the limbs, or other motor difficulties. Vascular dementia can cumulatively do great damage to a person's cognitive abilities, but each episode is discrete. One stroke is predictive of later strokes, but they are not guaranteed. We can also do something about vascular disease: We can take medicines to lower our blood pressure, aspirin and other drugs to thin our blood, change our diet to reduce complications such as diabetes, and so on. And with post-stroke treatment, victims can often recover many of their lost abilities.

About thirty-five million people worldwide have dementia, with direct and indirect costs estimated at $160 billion. As the world's population grows and ages, the number of cases of dementia is expected to double every twenty years to sixty-six million in 2030 and one hundred fifteen million in 2050. Most people with dementia are cared for in the home; nonetheless, it's a staggering statistic that more than two-thirds of all nursing home residents have it.

Alzheimer's disease is the cause of the majority of the cases of dementia. There are 5.3 million cases in the United States alone. The cost of Alzheimer's in the United States is estimated at $100 billion; by themselves, Medicare spends $40 billion a year and Medicaid $30 billion on this disease. Most of us fear Alzheimer's primarily because of its progressive and so far irreversible effects. Once we have it, there is no going back. Over the years we lose our short-term memory, then our reasoning and ability to plan. Our language skills deteriorate, and we struggle with reading and writing. Eventually we lose the ability to care for ourselves physically. But worst of all, we lose ourselves . . . our personalities and our memories, everything that makes us human. Medication can temporarily slow the pace of Alzheimer's, but so far nothing can halt its insidious advance and its terrible toll.

Life expectancy after diagnosis is an average of five years, but the full course of the illness may cover twenty years. Alzheimer's is devastating to the elderly: 45 percent of all Americans over the age of eighty-five have it, and it's the sixth leading cause of death in the country. Caregivers themselves suffer from high levels of burnout and stress-related illnesses. Family members, who spend an average of forty-seven hours per week with Alzheimer's sufferers, often suffer from depression, social isolation, sleep deprivation, and other problems. Doctors are beginning to understand that the most effective intervention in Alzheimer's involves treating two people, the patient and the caretaker.

If dementia (primarily from Alzheimer's but also from other causes) could be delayed by two years in those aged fifty and over, the number of total cases would be reduced by *two million* over the next forty years in the United States alone. Imagine the impact this reduction in cases would have on the quality of life for these individuals and their families and friends, not to mention the reduced burden to society in terms of cost and lost productivity.

HOW ALZHEIMER'S PROGRESSES

Alzheimer's, which was first identified by namesake Alois Alzheimer in 1907, is a progressive degeneration of the brain marked by the accumulation of both plaque and neuronal tangles. Plaque is created when beta-amyloid protein builds up in the spaces between nerve cells, interfering with neuronal communication and other brain functions. Tangles are created when the tau protein, which normally functions as scaffolding, begins to twist upon itself and create neuron-destroying tangles. A spirited debate rages between the "baptists" (for beta-amyloid protein) and the tau-ists. Snowdon's autopsies of two hundred and fifty nuns, for instance, showed a "far stronger correlation" between Alzheimer's symptoms and tangles than it did plaque. On the other hand, other research has implicated that the toxins present in some forms of plaque are murderous to brain cells.

Early on in every potential case of dementia there is a group known as the "worried well." Their occasional lapse in memory may be a prelude to something more serious, but most of the time it is nothing. Eventually, some people in this group will develop mild cognitive impairment (MCI). After a year, about 10 percent of the people with MCI slide into dementia, with another 10 percent succumbing each successive year. Yet some people who develop MCI never get worse.

If the person with MCI has Alzheimer's, these early symptoms are the result of plaque and tangles beginning to form near the base of the brain. The damage slowly spreads higher and deeper into the hippocampus and throughout the neocortex. The spread of Alzheimer's is measured on a six-stage scale. The early stages, when the damage is confined to a small part of the brain, are marked by mild memory loss but little or no cognitive decline. Middle stages, when damage has moved into the hippocampus, are marked by more memory loss and cognitive decline, including confusion and agitation. Final stages, when damage has spread into the neocortex, include severe memory loss and dementia and the loss of motor skills. Snowdon's autopsies showed that, of the nuns in Stage I and II,

22 percent had developed dementia; of the nuns in Stage III and IV, 43 percent had developed dementia; of the nuns in Stage V and VI, 70 percent had developed dementia.

Alzheimer's proceeds according to what is known as retrogenesis. The sequence in which capacities are lost is the mirror image of the developmental process in childhood. First come, last go. Last come, first go. Our reasoning and long-term planning skills are the last to develop and the first to go. Our motor skills are the first to develop and the last to go.

There are two apparent reasons for this. The first is the result of the tau tangles and the plaque. The damage from the tangles and the inflammation from the plaque appear to stimulate brain cells to try to regenerate, but instead the cells misfire and self-destruct. As a result, the most metabolically active regions in the brain—presumably, those involving higher thought—are affected the most. The second is demyelination. The loss of myelin, the protective coating on nerve cells, has the same effect as the loss of insulation on an electrical wire: Our brain signals become disrupted. With multiple sclerosis, for example, the immune system eats away at the myelin sheath in the spinal cord, disrupting communication between the brain and the muscles. Myelin slowly thickens over time, so the first parts of the brain to develop (the ancient brain structures related to basic functioning) have the thickest coating. The last parts of the brain to develop are the regions of the cortex related to higher thought, so they have the thinnest protective layers. As the myelin around nerve cells begins to fray, the newest regions of the brain with the thinnest layers show damage first. Even though the disease spreads from the bottom up, the damage presents itself most severely from the top down.

One day we will better understand these processes, but the end result is the same: With Alzheimer's, our brain physically decays. The autopsied brains of Alzheimer's patients often show an atrophy of 30 or 40 percent in brain volume. Our mind "walks backward" in mental development in the same steps—but in the reverse direction—that, as children, we walked forward mentally. Caretakers often complain that Alzheimer's sufferers are acting childish. They are right. A person with mild symptoms of Alzheimer's has the cognitive capacity of an eight- to twelve-year-old. A person with moderate Alzheimer's has the cognitive capacity of a five- to seven-year-old. A person with severe Alzheimer's has the cognitive capacity of an infant.

Understanding that the progression of the disease leads to greater and greater psychological immaturity may improve treatment for the sufferers and reduce the stress of the caretakers. Early in the disease, Alzheimer's patients may act like rebellious teenagers, refusing to engage or denying certain realities because they do not want to accept responsibility for their actions. They would rather claim the theft of something than to having lost it. *We are prepared when a nine-year-old throws a tantrum. We are much less likely to accept a tantrum from an adult—unless we understand that mom or dad has biologically regressed to the level of a nine-year-old.* The ability to socialize, to carry out activities, and to deal with frustration all slowly decline in tandem with the increasingly juvenile mind of the patient.

Like people of any age, Alzheimer's patients need affection, support, praise, patience, the ability to move about and play, and opportunities for social interaction. It does not matter if they do not interact well. Young children do not interact well with their peers, either, but they still benefit from being in a social setting. Because this decline is well-understood, it is possible to find "age appropriate" activities until the very end—as long as we map activities to the person's ever-declining psychological age.

In fact, some programs have successfully brought together children and elders with dementia who are close to the same psychological age. The greatest wins come when the adults are slightly ahead of the kids on the development curve so that they can serve as mentors for different kinds of craft activities. When they spend time with these youths, the adults show more constructive behaviors and engagement, and reduced frustration in comparison with other activities. The children benefit from the adults' superior long-term memory and better coordination, attributes that remain strong until the illness is very far along. Such programs need to be designed *very* carefully. For example, the adults need to have mastered the task at hand in advance and need physical reminders of the

Functional landmarks in normal human development and Alzheimer's disease

Normal development (approximate total duration: 20 years) — *Alzheimer's degeneration (approximate total duration: 20 years)*

Approximate age		Approximate duration in development	Acquired abilities	Lost abilities	Alzheimer stage	Approximate duration in AD	Developmental age of patient
Adolescence	13 - 19 yrs	7 yrs	hold a job	hold a job	3 (incipient)	7 yrs	19 - 13 yrs (adolescence)
Late childhood	8 - 12 yrs	5 yrs	handle simple finances	handle simple finances	4 (mild)	2 yrs	12 - 8 yrs (late childhood)
Middle childhood	5 - 7 yrs	2 ½ yrs	select proper clothing	select proper clothing	5 (moderate)	1 ½ yrs	7 - 5 yrs (middle childhood)
Early childhood	5 yrs 4 yrs 4 yrs 3 - 4 ½ yrs 2 - 3 yrs	4 yrs	put on clothes unaided shower unaided toilet unaided control urine control bowels	put on clothes unaided shower unaided toilet unaided control urine control bowels	6a (moderately severe) b c d e	2 ½ yrs	5 - 2 yrs (early childhood)
Infancy	15 mo 1 yr 1 yr 6 - 10 mo 2 - 4 mo 1 - 3 mo	1 ½ yrs	speak 5 - 6 words speak 1 word walk sit up smile hold up head	speak 5 - 6 words speak 1 word walk sit up smile hold up head	7a (severe) b c d e f	7 yrs	15 mo - birth (infancy)

Figure 7-1. Alzheimer's disease damages the higher centers of thought first and slowly spreads, causing an individual to regress in mental abilities to earlier stages in life. A person with mild Alzheimer's, for instance, falls back to the mental age of an eight- to twelve-year-old; a person with moderately severe Alzheimer's declines to the mental age of a young child. Understanding this process of "retrogenesis" may enable caregivers to better prepare activities in keeping with the patient's increasing needs and better cope with increasing emotional issues, which are no different than those of children confronted with circumstances they cannot control or understand. *(Copyright © 1984, 1986, 2000 by Barry Reisberg, MD. Reprinted with permission. All rights reserved.)*

correct sequence for the task; and the adults and children need to meet regularly to establish a personal bond. But well-designed programs have proved a benefit to the young at heart on both sides.

WITHSTANDING THE ONSLAUGHT

That our brain can withstand, for some period, the serious physical degradations caused by brain disease is illustrated by another of Snowdon's findings on a subset of the nuns. Of those with Alzheimer's symptoms, 93 percent also had some kind of vascular damage. Only 57 percent of the nuns with dementia had Alzheimer's disease alone. Only *one* sister had dementia as the result of a stroke alone. In other words, most of the nuns with serious dementia had physical damage from both Alzheimer's *and* strokes—including small, unnoticed strokes. If nuns had only Alzheimer's or strokes, they were able to offset many of the effects of the physical damage. Follow-ups by Snowdon and others confirm that dementia is most likely to occur when we are hammered by a combination of Alzheimer's and vascular disease.

Even more revelatory was the relationship between cognitive fitness and the underlying physical brain health of some of the nuns. If 70 percent of the nuns with late stage Alzheimer's (Stage V and VI) had symptoms of dementia, then 30 percent of the nuns with significant brain damage *did not*. Sister Margaret was in the 90th percentile for tangles but had little dementia. Sister Bernadette had severe Stage VI physical damage but no dementia. These two nuns had scored high in cognitive ability as youths and they had carried on busy and stimulating lives. They are part of a group called "escapees" because they showed few signs of dementia despite serious physical brain disease. Some of the nuns showed no brain pathology at all despite advanced age. They are part of a small subset of the population that shows a remarkable resilience to brain disease. People who reach the age of ninety without dementia are less likely to develop it than people who are seventy.

Conversely, those in early stage Alzheimer's should have had little to no dementia, but 22 percent *did* have such symptoms. Sister Maria had only Stage II, but she suffered from serious dementia.

She had emigrated from Germany with Sister Dolores when they were both young and they had achieved similar academic scores in school. Like Sister Dolores, she had begun her career as a schoolteacher. Unlike Sister Dolores, who went on to multiple degrees and responsibilities, Sister Maria suffered from serious illness and severe depression, both of which kept her from working for long stretches. Eventually she withdrew from teaching and worked as a seamstress. Only part of her career could be considered cognitively challenging, and that was sporadic. Also, depressed people are nearly twice as likely to develop Alzheimer's as other people, though it is not clear whether depression is a precipitating factor or a sign of early onset. As with Sister Maria, depression usually precedes dementia by many years if not decades.

These and other studies provide the answer to the question posed at the beginning of this chapter. Developing our cognitive vitality does not prevent brain damage. Rather, an investment in cognitive skills creates a compensating reserve that helps protect our mental abilities from brain damage.

THE BRAIN AND COGNITIVE RESERVE

Perhaps the most critical way to withstand the ravages of brain disease is to develop a cognitive reserve—additional cognitive capacity. The aspect of it that is physical is called a "brain reserve." Derived from our brain size or neuronal count (the number of brain cells we have), brain reserve is considered to be passive, a part of our lucky inherited draw. It covers all of the physical structures that add capacity to the brain or improve its efficiency. Brain volume is one of the correlating factors for cognitive health or dementia. Not because people with big brains are smarter but because a larger brain can suffer more damage and still have enough gray matter to function, offsetting cognitive decline. As a group, men suffer less from dementia than women because, in general, they have larger brains.

"Cognitive reserve" is considered active because it is impacted by our choices. It refers to the cognitive capability, including additional physical connections in the brain, that we can develop through education, engaging work, and other taxing mental challenges that we undertake in our lives. The statistic mentioned earlier—that there is an 11 percent reduction in the risk of dementia for each year of university education—comes from autopsies showing that the same amount of brain damage in someone who attended college resulted in lower levels of dementia than in someone who had not. Separately, Bob Jacobs autopsied brains to study the Wernicke area, which is the area of the brain particular to the understanding of language. He counted the number of dendrites, the tentacle-like extensions of the neurons that receive signals from other brain cells. Jacobs concluded that education increases the number of branches in the dendrites and hence the number of interconnections with other brain cells.

Here again, we face the question of cause and effect. Do people who have a greater cognitive reserve naturally gravitate to and succeed in education and high-stimulus fields, or do education and high-stimulus fields help develop cognitive reserve? Did Jacobs find more dendritic connections in educated people because people with enhanced inborn language skills tend to go to college, or because education helped develop these connections? Snowdon's studies imply the first, though most other studies support the second. Undoubtedly, people with very strong cognitive reserves likely have some inherent genetic advantage that provides greater neuronal count, but that advantage must be acted upon, positively or negatively, by the environment.

One of the most interesting and decisive studies in this debate involves London cab drivers, engaged in a taxing (as well as taxiing) profession that requires them to navigate one of the largest, busiest, and most convoluted road systems in the world. The cabbies' posterior hippocampus, the region of the brain responsible for spatial memories, is larger than that of most people. The longer a cabbie has been on the job, the larger the size of his or her posterior hippocampus. Even if we assume that the cabbies might have an inherent gift for navigation (they must pass a difficult test to get a license), the fact that this region expands with use indicates that an enriched environment provides numerous physical changes in the brain that improve the cognitive reserve.

People with substantial cognitive reserves are able to resist cognitive decline until the damage reaches a certain point, after which they decline more rapidly than others. A rapid downturn for the cognitively fit may seem counterintuitive. For an explanation, let's return to Mike. We assumed that his lifestyle gave him a 20 percent greater cognitive reserve than an average person. In his twilight years, Mike takes a test that shows he has a 10 percent cognitive deficit. It happens to be a deficit identical to another person who has no cognitive reserve. For the cognitive deficits to be equal, it is highly likely that Mike's underlying brain damage is more advanced than this other average person's! Remember, his reserve does not prevent brain disease but rather compensates for it. Once the physical impairment exceeds Mike's ability to offset it, the more serious underlying physical damage will cause his cognitive abilities to deteriorate faster than normal. His decline will likely start later than average, but it will accelerate more quickly. It might seem unfair that the most cognitively fit among us will usually fail the fastest, but the reverse is true: A cognitive reserve enables us to maintain the quality of our life until very close to the end. When we go, we go quickly.

MANY AVENUES PURSUED; ONLY ONE NOW WORKS

One of my favorite writers is Iris Murdoch, an English writer of Irish descent. Author of novels, plays, poetry, and books on philosophy, Murdoch was recognized as a brilliant and independent woman. The movie *Iris,* which contrasted her life as a lively young woman with her life as an aging woman suffering from the depravations of Alzheimer's, is enormously affecting. It poignantly reveals the manner in which dementia disintegrates our personhood—and also the enormous pressure it places on overwhelmed family members. Murdoch lived to be seventy-nine, and we can presume that her cognitive reserves must have delayed the crumbling of her mental faculties. That someone of her brilliance succumbed to Alzheimer's, however, makes it clear that no one is safe. Cognitive reserves do not prevent brain disease. They only significantly reduce the risk of it and—usually—delay its manifestation.

Of the various forms of dementia, Alzheimer's is the most fright-

ening because the disintegration of Iris Murdoch is the disintegration of everyone who gets the disease. Late onset Alzheimer's, the
variety that afflicts most of the population, has a genetic association, particularly with the class of genes called apolipoprotein E
(ApoE). ApoE is essential to the metabolism of certain lipoproteins,
which are complex structures of fats and protein that can function
as enzymes, can be used to build cell walls, and can help store energy. About two-thirds of us have the ApoE-3 gene, which appears
to be "Alzheimer's-neutral." About one in ten has ApoE-2, which
appears to help protect us from Alzheimer's but increases the risk
of cardiovascular disease. About one in five people have ApoE-4,
which increases the risk of Alzheimer's to three times greater than
normal. A percent or two of the population inherits the ApoE-4
gene from both parents, raising the risk to between eight and thirty
times greater than normal. Even so, the gene is not highly predictive—
roughly half the people who get Alzheimer's do not have ApoE-4—
so most medical practitioners do not call for genetic testing to see
who has the "bad" version of ApoE. There are likely other undiscovered genetic complications that contribute to the disease. They
must be common, because roughly half of us, if we live long enough,
die of Alzheimer's.

That such a large percentage of us carry several sets of potentially killer genes is—counterintuitively—the result of evolution.
Genes care only about making babies. If a trait helps us survive long
enough to create healthy offspring, then that trait will be selected
for, and it will spread through the population over the generations.
The benefit of the ApoE gene to our metabolism through our
child-bearing years (and beyond) biologically trumps the downside
of potential dementia, which normally appears long after we have
ceased procreation.

Our biggest concern about Alzheimer's is that it may not be a
specific disease treatable by some yet-to-be discovered medical intervention. It may be the accumulation of normal wear and tear, of
the oxidative stress and inflammatory processes we see with age in
many parts in the body. High levels of C-Reactive Protein, part of
the body's inflammatory response, are associated with dementia as
well as strokes and heart attacks. Unlike a worn-out hip or knee

joint or a damaged liver or kidney, we have no way to replace a failing brain.

A possible cure for Alzheimer's is likely many years away. So many different factors play a role: different genes located on different chromosomes, tau protein, plaque, strokes, general inflammatory processes, and so on. Studies of antioxidant vitamins, nonsteroidal anti-inflammatory drugs (NSAIDs), statins—even potential vaccines—have to date been contradictory or painfully disappointing. Folic acid, which is now added to certain foods, and lycopene, found in tomatoes, appear to offer some benefit. Snowdon found that 70 percent of nuns with high lycopene levels were alive six and a half years after an initial study compared with only 13 percent of nuns with low levels. Others have found similar positive results for both of these substances.

It is not clear whether lycopene helps lower the risk of Alzheimer's or is simply an indicator of good health, but regular servings of tomato sauce are a wise precaution. B vitamins may also help, but too much of any item is likely to trigger the body to counterreact. As for the rest of our diet, the best advice is that whatever is good for the heart is also good for the brain. We should heed the advice of our mothers and doctors and eat plenty of fresh vegetables, lots of nuts, fruits, and grains, minimizing our consumption of red meat and highly processed sugary foods. We should watch our portions. If we drink, it should be modestly—and with friends!

What we *can* do that will make a tremendous difference is to create a cognitive reserve by finding ways to constantly challenge our brains. With no cure for Alzheimer's presently in sight, a cognitive reserve is all that we can count on to help compensate for physical damage to the brain—whatever the cause. Exotic experiments involving stem cells, antibodies, and the injection of viruses into cells are under way with the hopes of improving resistance to the disease, yet the expected reduction in risk is no greater than what can be achieved today with exercise and mental stimulation! A cognitive reserve enables many people to withstand brain trauma and disease for many years. The goal is to live longer and die with our wits. And, of course, if we live long enough, science may find a cure.

We are about halfway along our path in the study of cognitive

DRUGS CAN SLOW BUT NOT STEM THE TIDE

Alzheimer's research has been slow and difficult. More than 400 pharmacological treatments are being explored, in addition to gene therapy and other approaches. The U.S. government spends about $640 million a year on Alzheimer's research, less than what it spends on breast cancer even though Alzheimer's affects many more people.

As of this writing, five drugs have been approved for treatment of Alzheimer's, though one is not actively marketed because of severe side effects. Three of the remaining drugs—Aricept, Excelon, and Razadyne—help preserve acetylcholine, a compound that facilitates the transmission of signals from one neuron to the next. The drugs interfere with the enzyme that breaks down acetylcholine, thus keeping the neural transmitter active longer. Peak effectiveness appears after thirteen weeks; by twenty-six weeks, the effect of these drugs begins to decline. The treelike nerve structure that carries acetylcholine throughout the brain continues to wither under the onslaught of Alzheimer's, accelerating the breakdown of cognitive function. The drugs present us with a terrible choice: Should they be used when someone's mind is still fairly sharp, to give them the best quality of life? Or later, to stave off the worst of the dementia?

Despite the decline in effectiveness, a number of doctors believe that the medications help patients remain cognitively ahead of where they would be without them. Patients are often prescribed one of the drugs for several years. (A generic equivalent of Aricept became available in common dosages in 2011.)

A fourth drug, Namenda, reduces the levels of glutamate in the brain. Glutamate, another chemical messenger, is highly reactive outside of cells. Trauma, through physical injury or Alzheimer's, can unleash glutamate and severely damage nearby neurons. Anti-glutamate activity can therefore reduce this collateral damage from cell destruction. For some reason, this drug works better for people whose disease is further along; doctors often stage it in after one of the cholinesterase inhibitors.

Because they do not treat the underlying causes of Alzheimer's, the current medicines will never have more than a modest impact on it.

reserve. In Chapter 6, we learned that developing and maintaining our cognitive abilities provides the only significant way of reducing the odds of dementia and delaying it for as long as possible. This chapter shows that developing our abilities does not halt the physical decline of the brain but enables us to offset it through the creation of a cognitive reserve. The next two chapters will describe the marvelous things we now understand about the brain's biology. We will see how the brain's capacity to adapt to almost any situation provides the mechanism for building new cognitive capacities. Challenging the brain does something biologically good for it.

===== LESSONS IN BRAINPOWER =====

- Alzheimer's disease causes a psychological decline as well as a functional decline. The childish behavior of an Alzheimer's patient is the result of the patient's mind deteriorating to the level of a child's.
- "Cognitive reserve" is the cognitive capability that we develop through education, engaging work, and other taxing mental challenges in our lives. Cognitive reserve does not prevent brain disease, but it can offset the *effects* of brain disease.
- By delaying dementia, we can reduce the burden on families and the cost on society; more important, we can enable millions of people to maintain their minds and their quality of life until the very end.

EIGHT

Lonely Neurons Die

Until the mid-1980s, one of the most advanced air forces in the world used a certain set of sensory motor tests to determine whether prospective pilots had the hand-eye coordination and reflexes to fly sophisticated fighter jets. It was believed that such skills were inherent in a person's physiology. You had the right stuff, or you didn't.

This assumption, and the tests that had been developed from it to screen thousands of applicants for the twenty or thirty available positions, were undone by a generation of pilot wannabes who grew up on . . . Pac-Man. The dot-devouring videogame, a cultural icon of the 1980s and one of the most popular games of all time, improved the hand-eye coordination of so many youths that the military could no longer use existing tests to screen for potential aviators. Too many people passed.

The positive effect of videogames on motor skills has since been documented many times. Compared to non-gamers, videogamers can process visual information more quickly; can track 30 percent more objects; can do a better job of tracking two different targets in two different locations; and are 20 percent faster in responding to visual and auditory clues. Such skills appear to be generalized, extending beyond gaming to general cognitive tasks. In one test, gamers answered general questions 25 percent faster than non-gamers, with the same accuracy. The ability to act quickly, especially in response to environmental cues, is equally valuable to someone flying a fighter jet in an enemy-filled sky and someone driving a car in a child-packed neighborhood. Such benefits need not coerce parents into allowing unlimited game time, however, because an excess of time spent gaming means that other skills that are at least as valuable are *not* being developed. Among other things, playing videogames after doing homework caused high school students to sleep more poorly than if they had watched TV. They also remembered less of their homework, possibly because the intensity of the gaming experience overrode the study topic.

In the category of art predicting life, the movie *The Last Starfighter* and the novel *Ender's Game,* both released in the mid-1980s, were based on the premise that videogames and simulations were used to train unsuspecting teenagers to fly spacecraft in galactic wars. Today, military organizations are among the largest buyers of game simulations, for everything from warfare to hostage negotiations to development of language skills. The main purpose of these simulations is to provide safe and inexpensive ways to train people to deal with confusing and potentially dangerous situations. Flight simulators, both professional and game-oriented, have long been used in this manner, helping pilots practice takeoffs and landings through bad weather and failing systems, without the concern of a real crash. Some games develop leadership skills by presenting participants with difficult choices such as being able to rescue some but not all of a group. In this respect, videogames and simulations primarily provide a large file of case learning so that the subject is unlikely to encounter a totally new situation during a field emergency. Games that focus on speed, however, have improved players' cognitive swiftness *and* their experience portfolio.

As with our London cabbies and their navigational prowess, gamers do not necessarily have better inherited reflexes than the rest of us. They gain improved hand-eye coordination and faster response times *through experience.* What's more, they are not "smarter" about game play, and they do not have better strategies for picking out one object from among many. They are just quicker. Most of us coordinate hand-eye movements in the parietal lobe of the brain. Brain scans show that experienced gamers instead use the prefrontal cortex to help coordinate these movements, presumably because doing so increases the physical control and speed needed for gaming. The brain recruited *an entirely new area* to aid in information processing. The highly addictive and oft-lamented video-game turns out to be an eye-opener when it comes to demonstrating how much the brain can change when given the right stimulation.

JUST ONE WORD: PLASTICITY

Neural plasticity is the formal phrase for the brain's ability to physically change as the result of new stimulation. Mastery of the simplest task or storage of the briefest memory requires change in the brain, usually in a small number of neurons. Plasticity, or cortical remapping, refers to wholesale changes in larger areas of the brain. As with the gaming example, parts of the brain normally used for one function can be recruited to handle another.

Our knowledge of plasticity comes from a series of studies relating to sensory inputs from the body. Many of these studies sound like bizarre science fiction stories: *The Ferret Who Saw What It Heard. The Musician Whose Fingers Froze. The Woman with Half a Brain.* Far from fantasy, they are legitimate studies that have overturned a hundred years of accepted scientific thought.

Scientists are able to map the locations where sensory inputs are processed in the brain, though these locations vary somewhat from person to person. Sensitive parts of the body such as the lips or the fingers have larger brain maps than less sensitive areas, and body parts that are close together are processed in adjoining parts of the brain (for example, inputs from the fingers are processed next to one another).The odds increase that one part of the brain will be recruited for another use if the processing areas are physically adjacent.

Animal studies conducted by award-winning scientists Mike Merzenich and Edward Taub, among others, show conclusive proof of brain plasticity. In one study, a ferret's ocular nerves were surgically removed and its auditory nerves were connected to its visual cortex. The ferret could see normally. The nerve from a monkey's middle finger was cut, severing its feed to the brain. The brain areas for the fingers on either side invaded the now-unused brain space, growing to twice their previous size. Prolonged exposure to white noise caused the auditory cortex of rats to rearrange; as a result, noise-exposed rats could hear better in noisy environments than typical rats but worse in quiet environments.

Human plasticity is equally remarkable. Musicians' brain maps vary according to the type of music they play. Finger maps in the brains of Braille readers are much larger than normal. Even more startling, they vary according to the level of the reader's exposure to Braille. Test subjects had the largest finger maps on Fridays, after the accumulation of a week of Braille training, and the smallest on Mondays, after the weekend break. Their brains recruit part of the unused visual cortex to help in the finger-based reading. Similarly, brain areas related to peripheral vision are several times larger in deaf people than in hearing people, enabling the deaf to more quickly and accurately detect moving targets off to their sides. In the absence of hearing, visual processing takes over the use of "abandoned" auditory cells. Mothers' brains rewire during the first months after childbirth; brain volume increases and other structural changes occur in areas related to maternal motivation. (Primate studies show that the same thing also happens to new fathers.)

Plasticity leads to extraordinary adaptations. A woman suffering from damaged inner-ear nerves had serious balance problems. Her tongue was fitted with a device that gave her a mild electrical stimulus on the front, back, left, or right side, depending on which direction she was leaning. The brain used these inputs to reinforce the fuzzy signals from the woman's inner ear, and she rapidly ceased to wobble. Blind people are able to sense objects by the way they reflect sound or change air movements; a blind boy who used clicking sounds to echolocate like a bat could ride a bike and play sports.

These studies, Merzenich's in particular, reveal an intriguing fact. During initial learning, the brain map expanded. As learning continued, it began to shrink somewhat. First connections proliferated; then they consolidated. Maps became more refined and detailed as the brain became more organized. Neurons fired faster. The better a task was learned, the more efficient the brain became.

How all these elements of plasticity add up is demonstrated by one case study, that of a woman who was born with only the right hemisphere of her brain. Her cognitive losses are minimal considering that she is missing her entire left hemisphere. Normally, the right hemisphere is involved with non-verbal communication such as facial expressions, emotions and emotional connections with others, and music and other artistic abilities. The right hemisphere is considered the "creative" side. The left hemisphere is responsible for speech, writing, and abstract thought. The left hemisphere is considered the "logical" and organized side. As most know, the body's sensory and motor nerves switch sides in the brain so that the right side of the brain controls the motor skills on the left side of the body and vice versa.

Not surprisingly, the woman's right arm and leg are weak, and her brother filches her French fries because her right visual field is blind. She struggles with abstract thought and gets lost easily. She is good, however, with concrete matters. She has savant-level calculating skills, and her hearing and sensitivity to touch are painfully acute. She reads, enjoys music, has a part-time job, and has fairly normal speech. As a child, her love of music was so strong that her father made her crawl before she could listen to it, a discipline which helped her learn how to walk. All in all, she is happy with her life.

All of these cases have emerged over the years in the scientific literature. Many of them, including the woman with half a brain, are collected in *The Brain That Changes Itself,* a book by Norman Doidge. Doidge celebrates the science, the scientists, and the patients themselves—some of whom assisted in devising solutions to their own cognitive impairments. He provides both a technical and human survey of the history of neuroscience and the study of brain plasticity.

Though "plasticity" generally means "malleability," our ability to learn a new task also means that any task learned too well can lead us straight to cognitive rigidity. Professional musicians, for example, use the same fingers together so much that they sometimes lose the ability to use them separately. The adjacent brain areas fuse together so that both fingers respond as one. The solution is to tape one finger down and force the use of the other one until the brain maps separate again. A similar thing happens to people with obsessive-compulsive disorder, whose impulses intensify over time through repetition, and with neurotics, who may become tortured by recurring unpleasant thoughts.

Though sensory inputs lead to new brain connections, we seldom recognize that thoughts have the same effect. Mental practice of the piano produces the same physical changes in the brain as physical practice. A person's actual performance will not be as good; but short real-world practice will catch him or her up to those who practice only physically. Infants light up the same part of the brain when they see an adult reach for an object as when they reach for it themselves. Their brain maps change through imagination! Many professional athletes watch replays of themselves during their best performances to mentally "tune in" to their top skills. Such preparation, along with practicing shots or goals in their heads, helps more than psychologically. It lays down the proper neural groove.

THE BIRTH OF PLASTICITY

Brain plasticity is so deeply ingrained in our biology that it begins even before birth. A huge surplus of neurons is created during gestation, peaking just before the neurons begin to differentiate. From this point until many years after a child is born, the brain goes through a cycle of neural pruning. This pruning is the result of "neural Darwinism," a term coined by Gerald Edelman, whose circuitous path through biology led to breakthroughs in both immunology and neuroscience. Edelman won the Nobel Prize for uncovering the structure of antibodies and for demonstrating that cells that produced the correct antibodies were preferentially selected for reproduction. This Darwinian response is what we need to fend off disease: rapid multiplication of the kind of cells that can kill off a particular kind of foreign invader, without our body having to maintain a huge standing army of every possible type of defender.

Edelman proposed a similar competitive principle that leads to the selection of the fittest neurons. DNA creates the gross architecture of the brain: the major sections and circuits, their primary functions, and the order in which brain-building unfolds. DNA is not complex enough, however, to map the entire brain of complex creatures such as humans. At the level of individual neurons and small groups of neurons, connections develop through a combination of genetic instructions, local biochemicals that affect the genetic coding, and interactions with the environment that are unique to every creature and every brain.

In humans, thousands of neurons per minute are produced in early gestation. The sheer number of brain cells and connections makes it probable that more than one area of the brain will develop the ability to respond to the same sensory inputs. An infant's ability to track and focus on a particular object, for instance, is likely to emerge in more than one bundle of neurons in the visual cortex. The bundle that works most efficiently will steadily accumulate more connections. The initial differences do not have to be great before a cascading effect results in one neural bundle intercepting and responding to the majority of similar stimuli, dominating the competition. Like a fast-food joint on a bad corner, a less competitive neural bundle will see traffic decline faster and faster, will lose its chemical ties to surrounding neurons, and will soon go out of business. The metaphor is apropos because in the marketplace this competitive phenomenon is labeled the "network effect."

Here we come to the underlying reason for the brain's plasticity: biological competition related to stimuli. Impoverished environments result in animals that have many fewer connections, and brains that are 10 to 20 percent smaller than normal. Kittens raised without visual stimulation had fewer and shorter dendrites and 70 percent fewer synapses in their visual cortex. When visual stimulation was limited in one eye, and then restored, the limited eye was severely impaired because the other eye had usurped most of the unused processing territory in the visual cortex. When the dominant eye was physically removed, eliminating the competition, the brain area corresponding to the impaired eye expanded considerably. These examples show how genes drive the development of the brain's primary structures but environmental stimuli and competition drive the development of the brain's finely honed structures.

Initial pruning in the womb accelerates as neuronal cells begin to specialize. During the final ten to twelve weeks of gestation, the number of neurons declines rapidly—as much as 70 percent. The process has two elements: neural pruning, a reduction in the number of brain cells; and synaptic pruning, a reduction in the number of connections. The fittest neurons and synapses form the pathways, the functional groupings, and the patterns of interactions that survive and thrive throughout life. This process of consolidation continues to occur throughout childhood with peaks at roughly one, three, and thirteen years. Children aged twelve to fourteen show a 25 percent reduction in the delta wave, a deep slow brain wave that occurs during sleep. Researchers take the shift to be evidence of the brain's reorganization. The changes relate to age rather than sexual maturity, though there is likely an indirect connection. Teenagers show a small loss of volume in the cortex; studies on rats confirm that the reduction in this phase of physical maturity is due to a loss of neurons.

As a result, the adult brain has 41 percent fewer neurons than the brain of a newborn. To a much lesser degree, pruning continues daily throughout life. It may seem scary to lose such a huge proportion of our brain cells, but we start out with many more than we need. These superfluous cells set the stage for competition. Something happens to us once or twice, and the brain stores the data away. Then nothing comparable ever happens again. The connection has little use, so the brain discards it, freeing resources for connections that matter. Pruning rids the brain of deadwood. Neurons that have strong, active connections survive. Neurons with few connections, including those that are damaged, are weeded out. It is survival of the fittest.

After so much pruning, what have we got left?

Only the most complex organ on the earth. Common estimates put the number of neurons in the adult brain at between 10 and 100 billion. The high side is equivalent to the number of stars in the Milky Way, a coincidence that charms commentators. A recent study using radioactive isotopes put the number of neurons formally at "86.1 ± 8.1 billion" in an adult male brain and slightly fewer, "84.6 ± 9.8 billion," non-neuronal (glial) cells. The study's exactitude must give us comfort, as well as pause. The "good" neu-

CONSIDER THE COMPLEXITY

Drosophila, the common fruit fly, has been the subject of uncounted scientific studies throughout the years. The fly's biology is complex enough to provide a comparison to larger creatures, including humans, but simple enough to be studied in depth. Recently scientists were able to map a good portion of the fly's brain, one neuron at a time. Using fluorescent green dye, they traced the locations of roughly 10,000 neurons of the fly's 100,000 total neurons.

They discovered a complex computer inside a tiny brain. The fly's brain has at least forty-one local processing units; six hubs; and fifty-eight gridlike structures. It appears to be a combination of a supercomputer like IBM's Watson and a distributed computing system like the Internet.

The human brain is 860,000 times bigger than the fly brain. How many CPUs, hubs, and grids is it likely to have?

rons, the active ones, can have between 10,000 and 30,000 connections with other neurons. A section of the brain containing a billion connections might take up no more space than the head of pin. Our brains have multiple trillions of connections.

Because most of the connections between neurons are local, we may wonder how the brain communicates in a coordinated fashion across such an immensity of cells. Imagine trying to cross-wire the Milky Way! MIT's Marvin Minsky has pointed out, though, that if a billion independent "agents" (a small number of neurons doing a single task) are connected to just thirty other small agents, there would be only "six degrees of separation"—six links—between any two agents in the brain. And instead of thirty connections for each agent, we often have tens of thousands!

A WHOLE LOT HAPPENS UNDER THE HOOD

What happens "under the hood" accounts for the brain's ability to remain plastic throughout life. A number of biological processes kick into gear whenever the brain is challenged with new experi-

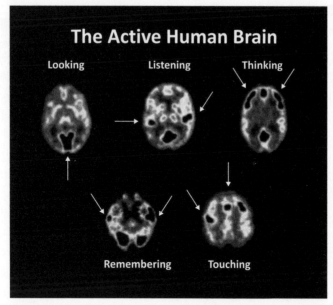

Figure 8-1. PET scans demonstrate that different parts of the brain become active with different tasks, as shown by the amount of glucose being metabolized. The more activity, the more glucose that is burned, corresponding in the graphic to the darkest regions for each brain. Because blood flow increases in the areas doing work, mental effort improves the brain's physical health by bringing in more nutrients and carrying away more waste products. Mental effort also increases the number of neurons and blood vessels, which improves mental capacity. Thinking causes the brain to gain weight! *(Graphic based on PET scans done by Dr. John C. Mazziotta and Dr. Michael E. Phelps of UCLA. Used with permission. All rights reserved.)*

ences. Responding to new stimuli actually changes its physical attributes.

I remember like yesterday the first time I saw PET scans of the brain in 1983. After years of depending on photos for research, we could finally see the brain in live action. The PET scan (Positron Emission Tomography) picks up radioactive dye in specially prepared glucose that has been injected into the subject. When the brain metabolizes the special glucose for energy, the PET scan highlights the active regions, allowing researchers to more precisely identify which ones are related to certain tasks and which ones are not performing properly because of disease or trauma. The scans also show that blood flow increases in the areas that are doing work.

The parallel between mental exercise and physical exercise leapt out at me. Blood flow to exercising muscles leads to muscle growth. Blood flow to exercising neurons must have a similar effect. Active brain cells steal the goodies—blood, oxygen, glucose, and other nutrients. Better circulation also increases the elimination of metabolic by-products. Waste removal is particularly important for someone who has plaque, glutamate, or other toxic materials accumulating in the brain. Cells with good blood flow become physically stronger and healthier than inactive cells. Mental effort equals better brain health.

This recognition was by no means unique to me, of course. Any number of scientists pursued the implications. Later studies confirmed that mental effort can improve the brain physically and spur plasticity. Mental training for rats raised brain weight by 5 percent in the cerebral cortex, with neurons developing 25 percent more branches and blood supply. Environmentally stimulated rats had a 15 percent increase in neurons after forty-five days and a *five times* increase in neurons after ten months.

Plasticity is aided by many subsystems within the brain, most of them chemical. The brain would not be the brain without the chemical bath that permeates its tissues. These chemicals have a myriad of functions: They affect the way in which genes unfold, leave scent trails that guide cell migration, assist in signal transmission, and regulate any number of other processes. One family of such molecules, the neurotrophins, affects the growth and survival of neurons. Foremost among them is nerve-growth factor (NGF). NGF plays a number of important roles in the cell. As its name implies, one of its functions is the stimulation of nerve growth. Its primary purpose, however, is to correct mistakes in cell activities.

In anything as complex as a cell, things are bound to go wrong. Most of the cells in our other organs routinely die and are replaced. The lining of our small intestine is replaced about once a week; the outer layer of our skin becomes new every thirty-five days; the cells in most other organs turn over in terms of years. But most of our brain cells are as old as we are. As with any complex machinery, maintenance becomes more critical with age. *The more active the neurons are, the more they secrete NGF. The more NGF they secrete, the healthier they become.* The more we use the brain, the more good stuff we get.

EXPANSION THROUGH LEARNING

The most common example of plasticity is dendritization. Dendrites, the input side of the nerve cell, are the treelike filaments extending directly from the body of the cell. They receive signals from the axon, the output side, which is usually a single, longer appendage covered with a series of myelin sheaths that resemble cylindrical beads. The axon terminates in a pod (usually one, sometimes a few) that sends electrochemical signals across a small gap, the synapse, to adjacent dendrites. The dendrite receptors are tiny spines, so small and dense that fifty or more protrude on a stretch smaller than the width of a human hair. It is the huge number of spines on each nerve cell that creates the enormous number of connections in the brain.

Just as the brain prunes for lack of use, so it expands with activity. Learning of any kind increases the number of dendrites, their length and branching, and the density of their receptor spines, reinforcing the neural pathways to create and maintain long-term memories. The strength and frequency of synaptic connections alter the shape, thickness, and number of spines, often within seconds. Some neurons can gain or lose 10 to 20 percent of their spines within as little as a few hours. The more difficult the task being attempted and the more successful the learning, the greater the extent of the dendritic rewiring. Dendritization is how the brain deals with new information. Because the electrochemical activity related to dendritic connections helps cells live, we can increase our neurons' chances of survival by challenging our brains with as much new information as possible. The more neurons that survive and thrive, the larger our cognitive reserve.

═══ **LESSONS IN BRAINPOWER** ═══

- When we first learn, the area of the brain being used (the "brain map") expands. As our learning improves, the map becomes slightly smaller and more detailed—better organized. The better a task is learned, the more efficient the brain becomes.
- Sensory inputs (something "real") lead to new brain connections—but so do thoughts (something "unreal")! Mentally practicing a task produces the same physical changes in the brain as physically practicing it. Imagination can change the brain as much as reality can.
- Biological competition among neurons leads to the survival of the strongest connections.
- Mental training (learning) increases brain weight, blood supply, and the number of branches that neurons have. Challenging as many brain cells as possible with new information increases the number of neurons that survive, increasing our cognitive reserve.

NINE

The Way the Brain Changes and Grows

Now we come to one of the most exciting discoveries of brain science. For more than a hundred years, since the writings of Ramón y Cajal, the father of neuroscience, the scientific orthodoxy has been that all brain cells are created before birth or within the first year or two of life. A dozen years ago, almost no one in the neuroscience community believed that the adult brain could produce new neurons. Even recent texts on neuroscience continue to repeat this traditional view. Today we know that adult neurogenesis is fact, not fiction. Indeed, it is a major factor in brain plasticity. Part of the adaptability of the brain comes not just from the reorganization and rewiring of existing brain cells but from the creation of new ones.

That neurogenesis has only recently emerged as the hot topic in current brain research is the sad result of the field having ignored the work of Joseph Altman in the 1960s. Using the same kind of radioactive marking techniques as later researchers, Altman not only identified adult neurogenesis in rats but also identified the paths by which new neurons moved from their birthplace in the middle of the brain to their final locations. No one found the work convincing. Scientists assumed that the migrating cells were the support cells, glia, rather than neurons.

Altman's case is an example of what happens all too often when a researcher makes a discovery that goes against the grain. Findings are met with disbelief if not outright ridicule. Research indicating that bacteria cause stomach ulcers was ignored for nearly a hundred years, because no one believed bacteria could survive the highly acidic environment of the stomach. Australian doctors Barry Marshall and Robin Warren eventually won the Nobel Prize for isolating the actual bacterium in 1982. The doctors who developed a series of sharp head movements as a treatment for vertigo were considered quacks until enough other doctors stumbled upon the same findings. It turns out that a common form of vertigo, benign paroxysmal positional vertigo (BPPV), is caused by the shifting of small, balance-related crystals in the inner ear. Sudden and properly sequenced head movements can shake them back into place. I suffered from debilitating vertigo about thirty years ago; abrupt turns would make me ill, and I couldn't use an elevator because the sudden starts and stops left me dizzy. At the time, doctors couldn't find anything wrong with me, so they said I had a virus. Eventually my symptoms went away, but I wish I had known of this treatment, which is now mainstream.

So it was with Altman and neurogenesis. It wasn't until the 1980s that Fernando Nottebohm confirmed adult neurogenesis in his studies of birds learning new songs. Shirley Bayer, an associate of Altman's, and another scientist, Michael Kaplan, both separately confirmed adult neurogenesis in rats. Later studies in the 1990s confirmed adult neurogenesis in non-human primates, and then Fred Gage and Peter Eriksson demonstrated it in humans. Finally, years after Altman's first experiments, it was accepted that adult brains for most if not all mammalian species can give birth to new brain cells.

A thousand new neurons may be born a day in adults, but half or more die within a few weeks. It appears that cell creation is routine, but the survival of the new brain cells relates directly to learning. A strong correlation exists between cell survival, the difficulty of the task that's being attempted, and how well the person masters the task for which this new cell has been recruited to learn. Neurogenesis also occurs in stroke patients for a short time after strokes and it appears to aid in their recovery. Antidepressants seem to stimulate neurogenesis, a finding that may help explain the manner in which they alleviate depression. (Prozac increases the number of cells in a rat's hippocampus by 70 percent in three weeks!) How the newly born neurons are involved in learning is not yet known, though logic supposes that they add more connectional capacity to the system. New neurons in the hippocampus, the part of the brain related to learning and long-term memory, might also play a role in connecting memories in time, since neurons that are born close together in time are likely to be wired together.

Immature neurons (neuroblasts) migrate from their birthplace in the interior of the brain to where they are needed; the exact mechanism is not understood. Once they are in place, their chemical surroundings switch on genes that cause the cells to differentiate into the specialized neuron type for that region. How the new cells learn to integrate with the existing neural circuits—which have been operative for years and years—is not known. That they do is well documented.

Consider the following example: Studies on adult mice show that new scents stimulate neuroblasts to migrate into the accessory olfactory bulb, which is a part of the brain involved in the sense of smell. Within two weeks the cells develop into adult neurons. The density of these new cells relates to the amount of scent stimulus received. Two things are worth noting. First, neural Darwinism is at work even here. The initial wave of migration is followed by competition that reduces the number of newly generated cells. Second, only a new and different scent—*something that needs to be learned*—will trigger the creation of neurons, their migration to the scent organ, and the successful integration of the new cells with the old.

Neurogenesis also gets help from a relative of nerve-growth factor (NGF). Another member of the neurotrophin family, brain-derived neurotrophic factor (BDNF), helps with the growth and differentiation of new neurons and the formation of long-term memory. BDNF plays a role in both normal neural development and adult neurogenesis. Stress's negative impact on our cognitive health is at least partly due to the way in which stress hormones suppress BDNF, which can result in atrophy of the hippocampus.

Unsurprisingly, low levels of BDNF have also been linked with depression.

PLASTICITY RELATED TO LEVEL OF DIFFICULTY

These insights about brain plasticity help us understand the importance of stimulation for learning and for brain health. The degree of our brain's plasticity is directly related to the degree we are being challenged. This is equally true whether we're trying to master difficult new tasks or information or to recover from a major trauma.

Traditional treatments for stroke victims all involve compensating for the abilities that were damaged or lost because of the stroke. Consider a patient who loses the use of his dominant arm. Usually we would help the patient become reasonably proficient in using his off-arm to shave, write, and complete other routine tasks. The parts of the brain related to these activities would be stimulated, but the damaged part of the brain would be ignored. Thanks to satisfycing, the acceptance of a "good enough" solution, the patient's brain would see no reason to expend the energy needed to overcome the trauma that rendered the arm useless. With this approach, the patient's dominant arm would never improve. Edward Taub demonstrated a radically different solution. If we forgo the traditional approach, and we *tie down* the patient's compensating arm for several hours a day, forcing him to use the useless limb, it will begin to regain function. It will seem to take forever, but persistence will pay. After a few months, the hand will start being able to make simple movements, then more complex ones. Eventually a significant amount of function will return. When the "good enough" solution is removed, the brain will seek optimal recovery.

Consider what is happening inside of the patient's brain: Under the stress of his efforts, his brain begins to reroute neuronal connections around the damaged area. Dendrites grow and new connections and cross-connections form as he begins to re-master tasks. Nearby parts of the brain are being recruited to replace the lost processing power, and brand-new neurons are likely streaming into the affected area to help with regeneration and new learning. Recovery takes time. Newborns need a year or so to learn to walk and several more to master other basic physical, locomotive, and mental tasks. Why would it take any less time for an adult to recover from serious brain damage?

Because the rate of cell production corresponds to age, younger people recover from trauma faster than adults, especially the elderly. With the right therapy, a young stroke victim might recover in a year. A forty-year-old or seventy-year-old might take ten times as long. Too often, we assume that the effects of a stroke are irreversible in the elderly, because the seventy-year-old often dies of something else within that ten-year span, or additional strokes cause more setbacks. But with enough time and determined effort, we can regain most of the cognitive brainpower we have lost. What is often judged to be the end of recovery is instead usually a temporary plateau during which the brain consolidates what it has recently learned. Even in cases in which constraint-induced therapy was not tried until more than eight years after a stroke, victims still showed an average of 30 percent improvement.

All of the mechanisms underlying plasticity involve challenging the brain. The more difficult the challenge, the more the remodeling that occurs. It's not magic, wishful thinking, or psychological musing. Learning—particularly of any tasks that require real concentration—physically adds capacity to the brain and helps to keep it healthy. The brain's ability to physically change as the result of stimulation is what allows us to learn. Computers will be more like the brain when they develop this capacity: when running software can change the wiring of the underlying hardware circuits as our learning routinely changes the wiring in our brains.

Plasticity is at the essence of brain function. From before birth to the end of our days, the dynamic duo of stimulation and competition drives an internal Darwinian war to produce the most competent and versatile neurons. The outcome is the most prodigious three-pound package of protoplasm on the planet. Though we share 99 percent of our DNA with chimpanzees, much of the divergence relates to the brain. Differences in DNA are usually described in terms of base pairs, the chemicals that anchor the strands of the DNA helix. The chimp cortex differs from the chicken cortex by two base pairs—by two complex sets of genetic instructions. The human cortex differs from the chimp cortex by *eighteen* base pairs. So near, yet so far away.

Dendritization and neurogenesis are the primary mechanisms by which the brain maintains its plasticity, mediated by blood flow, any number of growth factors, neurotransmitters, and very likely other still-to-be discovered mechanisms. Evolution seldom picks a single path, and future research may well unlock other interesting secrets of brain function. Though we know little about neurons, for example, we know even less about their companion glial cells. Glia is the white matter in the brain that supports the gray matter of the neurons. (Fittingly, the name means "glue.") Glia hold neurons in place, nourishing them, shielding them from toxins, forming the sheath around axons, helping to create new synapses, and repairing or removing damaged neurons. They are considered secondary to neurons. But it wasn't too many decades ago that scientists had no idea what the cortex itself did. Now considered indispensable to brain function and our humanity, the cortex was considered somewhat extraneous, or at least secondary, to other regions deeper in the brain. We may be in the same position today with regard to glia. Further, we gain more glia as we age. The only other thing we gain in our lives is experience. Though the brain has roughly the same number of glia as it does neurons, the cortex has nearly four times as many glia as it does neurons. It may be that the cortex's high-performance neurons require much more support than the other parts of the brain, or that glia have a more sophisticated role in memory and thought than is currently believed. We do not know. This is just one of the remaining mysteries about the brain.

That remains the refrain for the most interesting and difficult questions of neuroscience. "We do not know" or "the mechanism is unknown." For all that we have learned about the brain in the last two decades, neuroscience remains in its infancy. Anyone reading these words in ten years, never mind fifty, might find our current understanding as quaint as a modern physicist would find nineteenth century discussions on the "ether" that supposedly enabled light to travel through space.

We do know this: All of the marvelous mechanisms that underlie our cognitive abilities depend upon our actively engaging ourselves

STRONG BRAIN, WEAK JAW?

The human brain is roughly three times the size of the chimp brain, the result of genetic switches that trigger the brain to go through additional cycles of cell division. Sometime in the past, one of our progenitors must have received this mutation, benefited from it, and gone on to reproduce in significant numbers.

Yet our ancestors had small heads much like chimps. How did their brains grow larger without being crushed within their skulls? A possible answer comes not from a brain scientist but from a surgeon studying genetic problems in muscle-making genes. Hansell Stedman found a defective muscle-making gene in the oddest place: the human jaw. We have a physically broken variant of the primate gene for that muscle. As a result, the human muscle for clamping down the jaw has only one-tenth of the power of the corresponding muscle in an ape or a chimp. We're deformed!

At birth, a primate's skull bones are separate and flexible. (This is why some human babies have oddly shaped skulls immediately after being squeezed through the birth canal.) The chimp skull fuses very early, at about age three. Otherwise, their powerful jaw muscles would rip their skulls apart. Because of the weak human jaw muscle, our skulls do not need to solidify until as late as age thirty. They can expand significantly for decades.

We know that occasionally the gene switch controlling the reproduction of brain cells misfires in humans. When the switch shuts off too soon, it creates a condition called microcephaly (small head). With this disorder, the brain is roughly half of the normal size, often causing serious mental deficits. Neurologist Chris Walsh, who works with children suffering from this condition, has isolated the gene that is responsible.

Consider the reverse scenario. Several million years ago, some of our primitive ancestors developed the broken gene for jaw muscles, which marginally impacted their ability to browse and eat. (Perhaps it is even the reason they began to cook their food.) Along the way, one of them also inherited a gene controlling the reproduction of brain cells that stayed switched on too long rather than too short. The brain got larger. The skull could expand to accommodate it. Voilà, proto-humans took a giant step toward Homo sapiens.

Some scientists consider this scenario a plausible explanation of how intersecting mutations can lead to dramatic changes in a species. Others consider it far-fetched. If true, it will not be the first time that evolution has failed to run in a straight line. Our intelligence could stem from the left-right punch of the exuberant growth of brain cells and a busted jaw gene.

in the real world. The number of logical or artistic connections we make in our brains, the number of experiences we have and memories we create, directly relate to the number and density of the underlying physical connections. Neurons that fire together, wire together; neurons that fire apart, wire apart. So the saying goes. If neurons do not fire, they do not wire. If they do not wire, they go away. Use it or lose it. Neuroscience has adopted that popular expression. If brain cells have to die, we want them to be the ones that are not doing anything. But we would rather put all our brain cells to some kind of constructive work.

Maximum brainpower hinges on neurons being activated regularly, and regular activation depends on mental effort. Lonely neurons die. With their death our cognitive vitality fades. Connected neurons thrive. With their connections our cognitive reserve increases. Cognitive effort drives low-level biological processes that give our brains physical strength and our minds mental vigor.

===== LESSONS IN BRAINPOWER =====

- Adult neurogenesis—the birth of new brain cells in adults—has only recently been accepted as scientific fact. Survival of the cells, however, depends on how much learning the new brain cells are required to do. The more difficult the task that's being attempted, and the more successfully we master it, the greater the likelihood that the new cells will live.
- Compensation has been the traditional treatment for stroke victims. However, forcing a patient to try to regain lost abilities will usually lead to significant recovery. Effort stimulates the brain to repair or work around damaged areas.
- Learning—particularly any task requiring real concentration—physically builds the brain and helps to keep it healthy.

PART III

CHANGE AS A PATHOGEN

IF CHANGE IS SO GOOD, WHY DOESN'T EVERYONE EMBRACE IT?

TEN

Why Not Chase After Change?

If an engaged brain is central to our long-term physical and mental vigor, and if that vigor comes from constantly engaging the brain with new stimuli, then the best kind of life must be one that is full of change. Why do we not constantly seek change? The answer is stress. Just as the drag on an airplane increases with speed, stress increases with the amount of change in our lives.

Consider what happens to Dave, who goes through some not uncommon setbacks of middle age. In a single year, he gets divorced, moves from his long-time home to a small apartment, loses his job in the economic downturn, and suffers the death of a parent. These painful emotional experiences increase his risk of a major health breakdown by 50 percent, compared to the average for his age group.

There is a vast scientific literature on stress and its harmful impact. One simple test developed by Thomas Holmes and Richard Rahe more than forty years ago can predict the likelihood of illness according to the number of changes a person has undergone in the last six to twenty-four months—such things as marriage, the birth of a child, divorce, the loss of a job, and financial setbacks. The illnesses range from major ones such as heart attacks (the most obvious) and cancer (the least obvious) to minor ones such as the common cold. In studying more than 5,000 cases, Holmes and Rahe discovered that people who had led more turbulent lives were more likely to become ill than those with calm, ordered lives. The more severe the change, the more likely a person was to fall ill. The researchers weighed the stress impact of various possible life changes. The most significant change, the death of a spouse, received a weight of "100." Other events, ranging from change in marital status to financial reversals to minor traffic violations, had less impact and were given lower scores. Anyone who scored higher than one hundred fifty points in life changes had a 50 percent increase in risk for illness. Those who scored higher than three hundred points had an 80 percent increase in risk for illness.

Holmes and Rahe's next study, for the U.S. Navy, surveyed sailors to find out what had happened in their lives during the six months they were at home port. Based on the number of life changes, the researchers were able to predict which personnel would experience the most sicknesses during deployment at sea—including relatively minor illnesses such as colds. The beauty of this study is that it was prospective. Not only could the doctors relate change to health problems, they could also *predict* health problems based on the amount of change in people's lives.

Many, many other tests have since been developed to predict a wide range of psychiatric and medical diseases (for example, stress-related heart attacks). Tests developed for war veterans, hostages, and other people who have suffered from severe stress have helped researchers predict potential problems. Though the probabilities vary for different diseases and from study to study, all of the researchers reached the same conclusion. A number of life changes in a short period of time increases the risk for illness. The magnitude of the changes is highly related to how soon disease occurs and how serious it is.

What may be less obvious is that the change does not have to be negative. Let's wave a magic wand and give poor Dave a great year instead of a terrible one. He gets married, receives a promotion that takes him to a new city, buys a new house, develops new social relationships, and has a child. His *joyful* emotional experiences give him *exactly the same increased risk for illness* that his painful experiences would have! Even a wealth of new *good* things can overwhelm us. We can adapt well to one major change, but a clustering of change leads to problems. The impact is cumulative. There is no inoculation for stress.

STRESS: WE KNOW IT WHEN WE FEEL IT

"Stress" is one of those concepts that everyone understands yet no one can easily define. Though humans respond to stress in the same way physiologically, we all respond to different kinds of stress and different levels of stress. A loud noise that sends one person through the roof might be barely noticed by someone else. A new job that excites one person could terrify another. Some people enjoy airplane rides and others are reduced to tears. Because our emphasis is on the stress created by change, we will return to the original definition coined in 1936 by Hans Selye, who pioneered stress research. He defined stress as the "non-specific response of the body to any demand for change."

To a certain extent, stress is positive. In order to flourish, we need to function at an optimal level of psychological stimulation. Though that optimal level varies from person to person, we all suffer the same symptoms if under-aroused: We get bored. Boredom feels psychologically painful. Bored employees are roughly as stressed as overworked employees. Without sufficient stimulation, we tend to fall asleep. When we want to pay attention while reading a boring book or attending a boring lecture, we will often touch the skin of our face or lips with our fingertips or stroke our hair to make ourselves more alert. These fidgety behaviors are evident in any library. I once made a movie of these actions with a hidden camera. It was like watching monkeys grooming themselves. We need stimulation to stay awake.

"Eustress" ("good stress") is a word coined by Selye to describe stress that stimulates performance. The stress that precedes a major physical or mental competition helps activate our bodies and focus our minds so we can gather our resources and deliver our best efforts. Whether we are trying to run a four-minute mile or achieve a perfect score on a college admissions examination, preparation plus a bit of fear can be a productive combination. Eustress challenges us to develop our potential. External factors key us up rather than bring us down. But eustress still taxes the body just as any other stress does. We cannot "peak" for physical or mental competitions every day. We will wear ourselves out.

In evaluating the impact of stress, what matters is not the absolute level of stress but the *change* in stress from a person's baseline (the level to which he or she is accustomed). For someone who grew up in a large city, the blare and commotion is normal. For someone who is used to a quiet rural area with a traditional lifestyle, just being in a city can be extremely stressful. A person whose first major job is in a hectic, high-growth, 24/7 industry will consider a frenetic pace normal. A person who works in a quieter, slower-paced work environment, and then transfers into a high-growth industry, can suffer debilitating stress. One high-tech manager says that his major job is to teach new employees that chaos is normal so that they do not succumb to the disorder that is part and parcel of their industry. The analogy he uses is whitewater rafting. The rafter cannot tame the river in order to have an orderly and predictable ride, but he can use his training and skills to navigate it successfully.

Whether a new situation creates stress or eustress depends largely on our level of preparation. Eustress occurs when we believe we have a good chance at succeeding in the task before us. The stress that a well-prepared student or a well-trained athlete feels is considerably different than that of a student who slept through his classes or an athlete who skipped most of the season's conditioning sessions. The lack of preparation of the latter two individuals will be compounded by their *awareness* of their lack of preparation. Whether stress is good or bad depends on our perception of the control we have over the outcome and whether the outcome itself is likely to be positive. The anticipatory stress that most of us feel before a wedding differs from what we feel approaching open-heart surgery.

Some believe that the actual situation is less important than how it's evaluated by the person confronting it. Developed by Richard

Lazarus, "cognitive appraisal" posits that if we think we can manage, we are less stressed. If we do not think we can manage, we are
stressed even though another person might not be. Lazarus divides
cognitive appraisal into two phases. The primary appraisal is
whether an event is a threat or a challenge. The secondary appraisal
is whether we can do anything about it. Can we cope or not? The
outcome of the analysis determines whether the event causes major,
minor, or no stress. Lazarus's view was the prevalent theory for
many years, and there is no question that a cognitive appraisal is
involved in our reaction to stress.

However, taken to its logical conclusion, the concept of cognitive appraisal turns stress into a totally subjective affair. If a person
is in danger, in need, or under some duress, and he or she is *not*
stressed, then everything must be fine. This perspective is dangerous
because it could be used to justify keeping people in miserable conditions as long as they feel okay about it. Poor children in the slums
of Sudan and India smile more often than middle-class American
children. Does this mean they are better off living in such conditions? "Ignorance is bliss" is a phrase that's often used to justify
keeping the impoverished in the dark. If they do not know what
they are missing, they will not aspire to it.

This mind-set is extremely objectionable. We should fight ignorance and poverty irrespective of whether the end result is that the
poor might be more stressed by a better life. In history, the theory of
the "revolution of rising expectations" posits that the awareness of
better possibilities has driven most of human progress by encouraging individuals to take the risks necessary to improve their lives.

A strictly subjective approach to evaluating stress is doubly
problematic. Some people live in conditions that are abysmal by any
objective standard and they do not act pathologically stressed.
Other people have everything and kvetch all the time. We must seek
balance. Subjective appraisal is important and can help us deal with
stress; but there is also the question of reality. Let us consider the
difference between a clinical psychologist and a social worker. The
psychologist has only the subjective data that comes directly from
the patient. The social worker also visits the patient's house, meets

THE COST OF STRESS

- Forty percent of workers report that their job is very or extremely stressful and 25 percent view their jobs as the top stressor in life.
- One million workers are absent every day because of stress, and more than half of all lost working days from absenteeism are related to stress.
- Stress is now the number one cause of lost work days in Australia.
- Males are usually the subject of stress studies. A major survey focused on females showed that women with stressful jobs have a 40 percent greater overall risk of heart problems than unstressed women. Women who are worried about losing their jobs have higher blood pressure and cholesterol.
- Mental health issues are at the heart of 72 percent of long-term disability claims and 82 percent of short-term claims, according to the consulting firm Watson Wyatt.
- Stress is responsible for 19 percent of absenteeism, 40 percent of turnover, 30 percent of disability costs, and 60 percent of workplace accidents, according to the consulting firm Chrysalis.
- Healthcare costs for stressed workers are 46 percent higher than those of other workers, roughly $600 more per person.
- Layoffs more than double the chance of a heart attack and stroke for an older worker. A person who loses a job has an 83 percent greater chance of developing health problems.

with his or her family, and can detect any discrepancies between the objective and subjective situation.

WIRED FOR THE QUICK KIND OF STRESS

From an evolutionary standpoint, humans are still hunter-gatherers. Biologically we are the same people who wandered the plains for tens of thousands of years hunting for game and gathering nuts, fruits, and other edibles. The only stressors we faced then were directly related to our survival. Will that creature over there eat us, or can we eat it? Can we outrun the forest fire or ford the raging river? Humans either made it or they didn't. No one suffered from chronic stress by worrying day after day about quarterly results or the possibility of job layoffs or whether an investment portfolio would last through retirement.

As a species, our biology has evolved to deal with the immediate stress of life-threatening dangers. Whether we are dodging a lion or engaging in a fistfight, we are wired to deal with short, dramatic events. We mobilize, we run or do battle, and we "come down" afterward. We do not care about the long-term downside of stress if it saves our life today. Truth be told, until the last hundred years very few people lived long enough for chronic stress to contribute to their deaths.

Humans are not well equipped to deal with chronic stress, even if the stress-inducing events are relatively mild. Falling sales, unrealistic deadlines, disagreements with a colleague: All of these hassles trigger the same threat response as physical aggression or another bodily threat. If the brain perceives "danger"—real or psychological, it does not matter—it responds within milliseconds by pumping stress hormones into the system. A person who is tense for the entire workday, from nine to five, may also be tense from five to nine in his or her evening at home. Unhappy marriages have been around since time immemorial, but in traditional societies lifestyles are simple, the roles between spouses are well defined, and the struggle for survival occupies most of the time. Modern society brings the contradictory elements of long isolated hours at work (often for both spouses); fluxing roles between husband and wife; consumption-oriented lifestyles; considerable leisure time that needs to be filled; and children who need to be educated and entertained—as opposed to being put to work. Such elements add considerably to the stress inherent in any relationship.

Almost all of us are a little tense every day. Our bodies repeatedly kick into "fight or flight" mode, over and over, for months and years. The cumulative impact is overwhelming. Nothing in our physiology prepares us for this. Selye's research, beginning seventy years ago, showed that stress causes heart attacks, strokes, kidney disease, and rheumatoid arthritis. Subsequent research has implicated long-term stress in almost every ailment found in modern society.

THE INCUBATION OF THREAT

Perhaps the major manifestation of stress is fear, the emotion we feel as our body revs up to confront danger. Fear is, of course, an adaptation to immediate threats. How might we respond to longer-term fear, for example, while waiting for a job interview, a major surgery, or a university exam? Not well, it seems. University students preparing for major oral examinations scheduled months in advance showed higher levels of stress than airborne soldiers before their first parachute jump out of an airplane! After months of continued anxiety, the students' stress levels rocketed on the actual day of the exam. Surgery patients whose operations are scheduled well ahead of time require more anesthesia than those who do not need to wait as long.

To determine the relationship between time and stress, my team arranged an experiment in which we threatened volunteers with an electric shock. The subjects were wired with dummy electrodes, and we monitored their heart rate, respiration, and perspiration (much like a lie-detector test). Three sets of volunteers were told that the shock would occur in three, six, and twelve minutes, respectively. The clock was positioned within everyone's field of vision. At the last second, all the groups were told, "Relax, you won't get shocked."

All of the subjects showed a spike in stress when they first heard that they would be receiving a shock. Afterward, the three-minute crew's stress level started to decline. It had tailed off slightly by the time the participants learned there would be no shock. The six-minute crew showed the same drop (to an even lower level), but after three minutes or so their stress levels started to rise again until they were noticeably higher than at the initial point. The twelve-minute crew repeated the pattern of an initial decline in stress followed by a steady climb—until it was much higher than in the other groups.

These results, in which fear is incubated to higher and higher levels, have been replicated in other labs. When someone learns of an approaching, ominous event, stress continues to rise for about thirty minutes, at which point compensatory measures kick in to keep the body's heart rate within reason, though overall stress remains high. The brain becomes more and more involved in the threatening images and negative consequences of the dreaded event, while self-soothing mechanisms such as reassurances—"don't worry, all will be well"—tend to lose their effect. In general, the longer we know of a potentially bad event, the more it looms in our mind. Even if we can use the extra time to prepare ourselves, a longer period is more debilitating than it is helpful. This is another indication that we are wired for short, fast stress and not long, slow stress.

HOW STRESS LEADS TO DISEASE

Our immune system normally protects us from viruses, bacteria, mold, and other pathogens. Chronic stress compromises the immune system, thus opening the door to disease. Stress has a particularly harmful effect on lymphocytes, the white blood cells that are our bodies' first line of defense against biological invaders. The body produces white blood cells in the bone marrow and stores them in the spleen and thymus until they are needed, at which point they're released into the blood. When there is no infection, the blood has relatively few white cells; during an infection, it has many; and afterward, the level drops while replacement cells are being created in the marrow. Anything that slows the production of white blood cells or increases their destruction harms our ability to stave off illness, including cancer.

Barbara Anderson and other researchers at Ohio State University have shown that, among women with breast cancer, high-stressed women suffer a 15.4 percent greater breakdown of NK cells, a kind of white blood cells that attacks invaders, than low-stressed women. High-stressed women also have a 20.1 percent reduction in their response to gamma interferon, a natural substance in the body that enhances NK cell activity, and have a 19.8 percent lower response by T-cells, another type of infection-fighting lymphocyte.

High stress and major depression also reduce NK cell and T-cell counts in patients with HIV. A reasonable T-cell population serves as protection against seven common cancers associated with HIV, and a reduced T-cell population significantly increases the risk of these cancers. Stress damages the immune system in many other ways, as well. The University of California discovered that the immune cells of chronically stressed people were the equivalent of ten years older than the immune cells in people with the lowest level of stress. Stress increases the odds of bacterial infections such as tuberculosis and strep throat, and substantially worsens reactions to allergies.

High stress and depression go hand in hand in reducing the effectiveness of our immune systems. A year after a spouse's death, the rate of depression for surviving partners is four times higher than normal, and the probability of an elderly person dying within a year of a spouse's death is much higher than normal. While at work on this chapter, I learned of an incident that made this statistic personal. A friend's father became seriously ill. Shortly after, her mother began to fail as well. Each knew the other was dangerously ill. Because of the care required, they were being treated in adjoining rooms. When the mother died, the family decided to tell the father. His daughter said to him, "Dad, Mom's gone. You don't have to keep trying." He uttered a heart-rending cry, lapsed into a coma, and died seventy-seven hours after his wife.

GOOD FOR EMERGENCIES, BAD FOR REGULAR LIFE

Stress hormones appear to create most of the damage to the immune system. The main culprit is cortisol, which is produced by the adrenal glands. In short bursts, cortisol readies the heart, lungs, and muscles for action. It promotes healing and coats blood platelets to form a natural coagulant to reduce bleeding. It is also a prime regulator of the immune system. Acute stress also stimulates the release of NK cells, presumably as the result of one of the stress hormones. As part of the "shock" experiments described earlier, we took blood samples before and after the subjects were given the threat of an electric shock. Their fear (acute stress) increased the number of NK cells in their blood. It is when stress becomes chronic that these white blood cells become depleted.

Indeed, over a prolonged period, excessive cortisol suppresses the immune system, particularly NK cells and prostaglandins, which are hormonelike substances that help support immune function. It also promotes the production of LDL, the so-called bad cholesterol that, in the short term, helps repair cellular walls. This is quite useful if we are suffering from stress related to a bodily injury. Over time, however, LDL can accumulate in the gallbladder to form stones or attach to artery walls to form dangerous plaque. Cortisol can also damage neurons, especially in the hippocampus region of the brain, which itself controls the secretion of cortisol. The more cortisol we release, the more likely we are to release too much in the future, increasing the stress reaction.

Conversely, prolonged stress can exhaust the adrenal glands, leading to an "adrenal fatigue" in which our bodies begin to release too *few* stress hormones. With less regulation, the immune system can become hyperactive, increasing the risk of autoimmune and inflammatory problems.

If stress contributes to disease, it stands to reason that a reduction in stress should improve our odds against illnesses, even serious ones. This conclusion has been borne out again and again. In the Ohio State research, lasting more than a decade, women who received psychological counseling had a 45 percent *reduction* in the risk of breast cancer recurring. If it did recur, women who received counseling had a 59 percent *higher* chance of surviving. Counseling helped patients understand the relationship between stress and cancer, taught them strategies to reduce stress in their lives, and helped improve communication with their doctors.

IMPAIRMENT OF COGNITIVE FUNCTION

Stress not only degrades our health. It also impairs our cognitive function. A topical example is the craze among young people for multitasking. If a young adult or young professional is not simultaneously texting, Facebooking, tweeting, blogging, listening to music, and watching YouTube, then that person is definitively uncool and supposedly unproductive. (Half of all students watch TV or browse the Internet while doing homework.) The presumption that every worker has instant access to a digital device is also making multitasking more and more of a necessity at work. The belief is that multitaskers are accomplishing more tasks, and faster, than their stick-in-the-mud colleagues who insist on concentrating on one thing at a time.

In actuality, multitaskers are reducing their brainpower.

Part of the problem is generational ignorance, the belief by each new population cohort that they are the first to discover everything from ethics to romance to technology. Throughout history, all bustling industries have engaged in multitasking in the general sense of the word—juggling many responsibilities at once, acting and reacting quickly, and making a number of important decisions under time constraints. The word "multitasking" took on its current use during the rise of the computer industry, when companies boomed and collapsed with equal speed and industry leaders were repeatedly being overthrown. The pace kept accelerating to "Internet time" and ever more rapid change. What has been lost in the mists of history is that the savvy multitaskers of earlier eras were all experts. Having worked in the same industry for many years, they were able to call upon their vast expertise to solve difficult questions quickly and efficiently.

Flash-forward to today's youth. They are not using multitasking to juggle their duties or to make quick decisions on the basis of a huge base of case-knowledge. Rather, they are attempting in school and at work to *learn* through multitasking. The belief is that they can assimilate more knowledge by making "quick cuts" across a vast range of information than by plodding through a single subject. Objective tests show, however, that this approach to building brainpower is a disaster.

Assuming that these high-tech whizzes would turn out to have splendid focus and control over mental abilities, Stanford researchers were shocked to discover that multitaskers were uniformly bad at just about every mental task. They were far more distracted by irrelevant items, had worse memories, and were slower at *switching tasks* (!) than non-multitaskers. By training themselves to constantly move from one stimulus to the next, they had developed the attention span of a dog on meth.

These results are by no means isolated. Vanderbilt University researchers found that doing two things at once slowed test subjects by one second on fairly simple tasks. The Institute of Psychiatry at the University of London showed that the IQ of workers who were distracted by email and phone calls fell twice as much as that of marijuana smokers. In general, it takes between fifteen and twenty-five minutes for people to recover from distractions and return to their original tasks.

Efforts to multitask are thwarted by the brain's basic mechanisms. Humans form one kind of memory when we pay close attention and another kind when we pay only partial attention. Learning a task through sustained concentration fires up the hippocampus, leading to the formation of a "declarative memory." This kind of memory, which requires full attention on the event, can be applied to other, unfamiliar situations. Learning a task while distracted, however, causes the memory to form in another part of the brain, the striatum. This kind of memory, called a "habit memory," is related to very specific tasks and is not easily transferred to new situations. People who learn without distractions have a much higher success rate in applying knowledge to new problems than do people who suffer from distractions.

In addition, the brain hits a bottleneck when it's forced to respond to several stimuli at once. As with computers, switching context creates overhead. One reason hearkens back to our basic biological wiring. Each time the brain perceives a new stimulus, it must first decide: useful or not? (In prehistoric times, the question was: friend or foe?) Change brings stress, so the constant effort to switch tasks causes the release of cortisol and adrenaline which, in addition to their long-term negative effects, also hamper the formation of short-term memory.

It seems strange that a culture seeing more and more attention-deficit disorder in its youth should encourage activities that cause distraction. The chronic inability to focus—what William James called the "extreme mobility of attention" and the "gray chaotic indiscriminateness" of the unfocused—has traditionally been viewed as the hallmark of an immature mind. The stress of multitasking overwhelms whatever value may accrue from a constant, superficial scanning of vast quantities of information. In practical terms, multitasking is nothing but a way to mess up more than one thing at a time.

Multitasking is a microcosm of the change that's inherent in modern life. Change brings stress. Stress is bad for us, both for our bodies and for our minds. We see that eliminating stress improves our health. So what happens when we are confronted with stress? As we see in the next chapter, our first reaction to stress is often not to deal with it, but to wish it away.

═══ LESSONS IN BRAINPOWER ═══

- Stress has such a powerful and consistent effect that we can predict the likelihood that a person will become ill based on the number of recent changes in his or her life. Too much positive change can be just as bad as too much negative change!
- Too little work can create almost as much stress as too much work because the brain requires a certain level of stimulation to be properly engaged and functioning.
- The impact of stress depends more on the *change* in stress from a person's typical level rather than on the absolute stress level.
- Whether stress is good or bad depends on our perception of the control we have over the outcome and whether the outcome itself is likely to be positive. If we think we can manage, we feel less stress.
- The longer we have to think about a threat, the greater our fear and the greater our level of stress.
- Humans are wired to deal with the immediate stress of life-threatening dangers, not the long-term stress of today's life. The biological mechanisms that prepare us for "fight or flight" wear out the body physically over time.
- Stress hormones damage disease-fighting white blood cells and other parts of the immune system. Reducing stress reduces the risk of illness and helps improve the chances of recovery from sickness.

ELEVEN

Denial of Stress

Because stress is bad for us, we tend to deny its existence. The most common and primitive way to cope with stress is to not think about it at all. This response occurs at the institutional level as well as the personal. Until the 1970s, the medical community encouraged denial in patients who were suffering from serious or terminal illnesses. Rather than tell patients they had cancer, doctors would invent things to say such as, "You have a fungus on your liver, but we can treat it." Or, "You have nothing seriously wrong, but be sure to come back to the hospital for chemotherapy and radiation." They used all kinds of misinformation in an effort to "spare" their patients, when in reality they were just sparing themselves the stress of dealing with traumatized patients. One justification used at the time was that people would become depressed if they knew the true nature of their condition. In fact, the frequency of suicide in people with serious illnesses is higher among those who have been painted a rosy picture than among those who are fully informed.

Everyone played the game: doctors, relatives, friends. For seriously ill patients, anxiety increased because of the disconnect between what they were being told and what they could see for themselves, including visits from teary relatives and the physical evidence of their own decline. They had no one to confide in and no outlet for serious discussions about life and death.

My mother died of cancer, and our family experienced this "speak no evil" approach. I became a very vocal opponent. Eventually, the Israeli Cancer Association asked me to help develop a more rational policy on what doctors should tell patients, which brought together contributions from a number of professionals, including young doctors who had studied in America and had witnessed better methods of handling doctor-patient communication. The new approach called for doctors to lay out the situation for their patients honestly but compassionately, providing them with a realistic prognosis and realistic estimates about the efficacies of various treatments—or no treatment. Doctors would provide the terminally ill with the psychological support and the time they needed to come to grips with their mortality and say goodbye to loved ones. These guidelines injected common sense and humanity into the process, ending doctors' efforts to avoid their own stress at the cost of their patients'.

If the medical community, which includes some of the most educated and rational people in the world, worked so hard to avoid the truth, I wondered, how deeply embedded in our psyches is the denial of stress? How do people deny stress? What is the result of that avoidance? This was in the early 1980s, and the concept of stress denial had not been systematically studied by anyone before. These questions led me to organize a major conference, the first of its kind, and I followed up with a book on the topic. My research showed that there are seven major ways in which we deny stress, all of which we use to convince ourselves that we need not worry about the underlying stress-inducing problem. They are:

1. Denial of personal involvement: It cannot happen to me.
2. Denial of urgency: It can happen, but not for a long time.
3. Denial of vulnerability: If and when it does happen, I can cope with it.
4. Denial of anxiety itself: I know something is happening, but I am not worried.
5. Denial of emotion: I acknowledge my emotion, but I deny its

source. I explain it away. If I suffer from a racing heart, it's because I have been exercising.

6. Denial of threatening information: I filter the information so that I do not perceive any threat.

7. Denial of all information: When presented with the truth, I deny it exists (often by a physiological reaction such as fainting).

A stressful event might send us to one form of denial, or we might go through several of them as more information begins to leak through our defenses. A smoker might deny the possibility of developing lung cancer. When confronted with statistics, he might admit that cancer is a possibility but dismisses the danger as something that will happen in the distant future (he will, of course, have quit smoking long before then). If any symptoms of smoking-related illness develop, he will deny any concern. That cough? It's just a cold.

Fainting is one extreme example of how we might deny stress in an emergency situation. Bad news creates such a shock that vascular constriction literally squeezes blood from the brain. Unconsciousness temporarily protects us from the implications of what we have learned. When we come to, we are surrounded by people who care for us, buffering the emotional pain.

Denial of stress is itself a strange phenomenon, for it involves the brain knowing something and not knowing it at the same time, what is known among philosophers as "middle knowledge." The paradox is that if we are afraid to think of something because its implications frighten us, we must have thought about it enough to have become frightened. This contradiction offers further proof that the brain has multiple levels of information processing—one that is conscious and at least one that is not. Enough information must cross the threshold in order to trigger a threat response that prevents further data from crossing through. We may process just enough to begin feeling tense or anxious without knowing why, and then our defenses go up without our conscious realization. Patients who are severely ill, for example, can pick up on all manner of clues about the true nature of their condition from the behavior of the people around them. But while they are not fooled, they do not necessarily want to confront the truth either.

The brain reacts to—and defends itself from—unpleasant ideas at an unconscious level. In a typical test, a word is flashed in front of test subjects so fast that they can perceive it subliminally but not consciously. The time exposure is extended by a few milliseconds at a time until the word crosses the threshold into awareness and the subject can read it. Fear-inducing words ("murder," "blood," "death," and so on) take longer for the brain to process than neutral words ("paper," "tomato," "desk," and so on). The moment we see a word with an obviously negative connotation, we try to block it out for as long as possible. It is an automatic, primitive way of postponing bad news for as long as possible. The brain must unconsciously be weighing the negative word to determine whether it poses any real threat. Subliminal images of a skull and crossbones every ten frames have been shown to increase tension in Hitchcock movies, as would the Nazi swastika for Jewish viewers. Symbols, rather than words, seem to have the greatest impact subliminally, perhaps because they require less interpretation.

Our ability to perceive information subliminally is the basis of the false belief that subliminal advertising can increase product sales. The original claim, that a movie theater was able to boost sales of soft drinks and popcorn in 1957 by flashing subliminal messages across the screen, turned out to be bogus. Later studies showed that such messages do not create a compulsion to buy. The fears of subliminal advertising were so strong, however, that the Federal Communications Commission banned it just to be sure.

In any event, for the denial of stress to occur, we must assume we have the ability to respond to subliminal information, and that it has the ability to shape our perceptions and memories. I once did a study (unpublished) in which the test subjects—a group of young adults, half men and half women—read a biographical passage supposedly written by a woman the same age as they. The story was about how she discovered a lump in her breast; it described her thoughts and emotions as she waited for the results of a biopsy. The passage also contained a lot of irrelevant details about her preference for clothing, shoes, certain colors, and so on.

Afterward, the readers were tested on what they recalled from the story. The male students remembered all aspects of the passage equally well (or not). The female students, however, remembered very well the aspects of the story that *differentiated* themselves from the woman facing cancer; for example, if she dressed differently than they did. They remembered very poorly those aspects of the story that had them *identify* with the woman; for example, if she liked the same types of food as they did. They were unconsciously distancing themselves from the threat of breast cancer.

WHEN DENIAL MAY BE OF VALUE

Roughly half of all cancer patients put off a visit to the doctor because they are afraid they have cancer! Ten percent of people who are clinically obese feel that their weight is fine and that they are in overall good health. Not wanting to face the truth is a strange excuse for people to avoid diagnosis and treatment. If denial of stress can kill by enabling such poor decisions, then why do we have such a deeply rooted mindset? It turns out that denial *does* have a benefit in acute, immediate stress rather than in chronic, long-term stress. Denial helps when the trauma the person is facing is so dramatic that it has to be cushioned.

Among the survivors of major floods and earthquakes, those who spend the hours following the catastrophic event walking around in a daze, seemingly unable to comprehend what's happened, tend to fare better in the long term than those who immediately grasp that their world has been destroyed. People who have suffered serious heart attacks do better if they are not fully aware of what has happened to them. Denial can help bridge the initial period of total destruction. The brain protects us from bad news by spreading it out over time, lessening the impact.

Besides being useful in dealing with the fallout of difficult or devastating situations, denial can also be effective when we are totally helpless, with no way to ease the stressful situation. Most stressful situations, however, are not life-threatening, and denial can be highly detrimental if it causes a situation to worsen until it *is* life-threatening.

COPING WITH STRESS

We deny stress because we fear that we cannot cope with bad news. In reality, coping actually requires less energy and is more successful over the long term than denial. We only have to *believe* we can cope before we start to make headway. Successful coping begins when we start generating positive expectations that things will turn out okay. Entire books have been written on techniques for coping with stress, so here we will focus on the fundamentals. The most critical distinction is between two types of coping: *problem*-focused coping and *emotion*-focused coping. The distinction between these two approaches to resolving stress, proposed by researchers Richard Lazarus and Susan Folkman, is widely accepted.

Problem-focused coping involves identifying the underlying situation that's causing the stress and attempting to resolve it. If the stress is being caused by work, problem coping would motivate us to analyze our time efficiency, prioritize our projects and tasks, form teams to deal with critical problems, and so on. If the stress is being caused by illness, problem coping would motivate us to visit a doctor, research everything about our illness, seek a second or third opinion, plan a treatment schedule, and otherwise become immersed in the practical issues pertaining to the illness.

By contrast, emotion-focused coping involves dealing with the emotional fallout of stress—by seeking social support, assistance, counseling, and possibly medication to aid with depression, engaging in stress-releasing activities such as sessions in the gym, and undertaking any other activities that reduce the impact of the stress.

The American ethos of "controlling your destiny," which puts a great premium on problem solving, tends to view problem-focused coping as the more appropriate strategy. However, this approach can compound stress when the source is unavoidable and cannot easily be handled. In a down economy, which prevents people from easily switching jobs, a problem boss is one example. Terminal disease is another. Asian cultures, in contrast, set more store on acceptance than on active coping. Depending on the circumstances, it's usually most effective to engage in both types of coping. If we are having trouble at work, for instance, we might apply problem coping first in order to reduce our stress and apply emotional coping second by seeking the support of friends and family in order to handle the stress that inevitably remains.

In many stressful situations our emotions can become so overwhelming that practical activity—problem-focused coping—becomes impossible. In these cases it is best to first use emotion-focused coping and then proceed with problem-focused coping. A good example relates to fighter pilots and the question of when they should abandon a plane that gets out of control. On the one hand, pilots are told, "Save yourself first, don't try to save the plane." On the other hand, if they ignore this directive and recover control of their plane at the last instant, they do not get a lecture for endangering themselves. Instead, they are celebrated for their flying prowess, and for saving the lives of the people on the ground and a multimillion-dollar aircraft.

These mixed messages cause a major dilemma. Imagine a pilot in the cockpit when an emergency occurs. Red lights are flashing, warnings are blaring, and altitude is winding down. The pilot has time to try only two or three procedures. If they do not work, he must eject. In the past, pilots became so stressed about whether and when to eject that they could not decide what to do in the few moments they had to save the plane. They would typically try the same thing over and over again, even if it was ineffective. I counseled the Israeli air force that they must train their pilots to be very systematic. Having a clear directive about when to abandon their planes would reduce the pilots' stress. In essence, all of their important decisions would be made on the ground before the flight. The air force's solution was to set a minimum altitude as the ejection decision. When the plane reached that altitude, the pilot had to abandon ship, no matter what. Having an unambiguous rule reduced the emotional response to the emergency. Pilots were able to think more effectively, increasing their odds of saving the plane. Here is a classic example of treating the emotion first and the problem second.

A common form of emotion-focused coping is social support. To benefit from it, we must spend time and effort investing in a social network of family and friends *before* the stress experience. We need to be able to ask for support when the time comes. Supporting others is a great way to reduce our own stress and anxiety, too, as another defense-related anecdote shows. In May 1967, before the Six-Day War, there was serious fear in Israel that cities would be bombed by the Egyptian air force. The government established bomb shelters and began training people how to behave in them. As in England during World War II, bomb-shelter wardens were selected to gather people into the shelters and keep them calm during air raids. I prepared the instructions for these wardens on how to deal with extremely stressed and panicky people. The best advice we could give was this: Find someone else who's even more scared, such as a child, and tell the stressed-out person, "You are responsible to calm down this little kid." Nothing helps us overcome our own fear and anxiety more than being responsible for someone who is presumably more vulnerable than we are. Instead of rushing to soothe people who are freaked out, thereby reinforcing their fear, we give them responsibility. It works wonders.

FIND WAYS TO DECLARE VICTORY

Understanding how the mind perceives stress can help people in a variety of leadership positions. Businesspeople cannot simply pile more and more work onto their support staff during tough economic times with the expectation that they will work even harder. If the load exceeds their belief in what they can do, output will collapse. People need to have a goal to strive for, some measurable kind of victory, even if they have to pick up where they left off shortly afterward. There must be something that enables the mind to say "we won." Such a victory might be a paid day or afternoon off, a pizza celebration of some milestone, a modest bonus, or something as simple as sincerely meant public recognition. Remember, productivity went up in the United States during World War II when workers were given Sundays off. Employees cannot march through hard times indefinitely. And the most important thing that employers can do to motivate employees during bad times is to be honest with them. The lack of information can be a psychic killer, as the next chapter demonstrates in detail.

ALLEVIATING STRESS AT WORK

We can all benefit from some simple steps to avoid unnecessary stress and maximize our mental energy during the workday. Here are a few tips:

- Begin with a quiet, brisk walk, which is excellent for thinking. The location should be familiar, to avoid the distraction of new outside stimuli.
- Don't carry a cellphone. Let the mind wander, always trying for the big picture, not the details. This can be the best and most important part of the day.
- Chat with someone over breakfast or coffee about the day ahead. After the free-floating thoughts of the walk, the discipline that comes from talking helps organize the mind.
- Do not begin the day with meetings. Take time to organize. Do a quick review of emails, deleting the less important ones and leaving the meaningful ones for later. Set specific times to review messages during the day—do not fall victim to constant digital interruption.
- Have times when the door is open for anyone to come in unannounced, but also have times when the door is closed for private thought.
- Despite the pressure to instantly respond to business issues, try to postpone even the most urgent matters to allow for quiet reflection. Even a couple of hours can make a difference.
- Use the lunch break to disconnect from the morning's problems. Discuss issues totally unrelated to company matters. In every country there is always the opportunity to complain about the government's latest actions.
- In mid-afternoon, stop to read an article related to your profession or industry but not specific to your company. This typically starts a new train of thought that will connect eventually with something you are working on.
- At the end of the day, spend time with family or friends, preferably not talking about work. Become immersed in something different and engaging such as music or reading. The fresh perspective helps reset the brain for tomorrow's challenges. Meanwhile, all the connections that you have made during the day are working away in the unconscious.

> • Throughout the day, take care to remember Lord Chesterfield's admonition: If we do one thing at a time, there are enough hours in a day to deal with every problem; but if we try to do more than one thing at a time, there are not enough days in a year to get anything done. By not becoming a slave to reactivity, and by dealing with matters without rushing, we avoid excess stress.
>
> Less stress means more creativity and originality.

A similar sort of approach might be used by politicians. Political leaders who want to guide their constituents through a major shift in policy must make a compelling case, breaking it down into simple, understandable, and manageable steps. The scope, complexity, and cost of American healthcare reform are intimidating, given our universal phobia of change, and this was compounded by supporters' less-than-stellar job of explaining its benefits. Even though the legislation passed, the anxiety surrounding it led to a significant drop in support—even among those groups, primarily working-class citizens, that would most benefit from it.

Change, and the stress it creates, forms a vicious circle. Once a set of changes rocks us, our ability to cope with subsequent changes also diminishes. It is no surprise that people abhor change because they realize it is distressing and difficult. We are conservative because the change that's needed for the health of the brain has its downsides.

As a result, we learn to avoid stress—change—as much as possible. This is particularly true of older people, who may not have the physical and psychological resilience of youth. We can counter our inherent conservatism, however. In the next chapter, we see that there is hope when we apply our full brainpower to managing stress.

═══ **LESSONS IN BRAINPOWER** ═══

- The most common way to deal with stress is to deny the existence of whatever is causing the stress—to wish it away.
- Denial of stress illustrates the strange phenomenon of the brain knowing something and not knowing it at the same time. Enough information gets through to cause us to put up our defenses without our conscious awareness.
- Denial of stress helps us survive catastrophes or helpless situations, but it can make lower-stress situations worse.
- Coping usually works better than denial. We can cope directly with the underlying problem or with the stress it causes. Often, we must first deal with the emotions caused by the stress in order to deal rationally with the underlying issue.

TWELVE

The Healing Power of Hope

The impact of stress is a common topic. My particular interest is its effect on our cognitive vitality. A method for testing this came to me after reading *The American Soldier* by Samuel Andrew Stouffer. Part of the book was about American B-17 aircraft crews in World War II. It was not until late in the war that allied fighter aircraft developed the range to accompany the huge formations of bombers flying from England all the way to their targets deep in Europe. Once the fighter escorts had to turn back, the bombers became extremely vulnerable to enemy fighters. Many were shot down. Crew members lost their comrades one by one, or plane by plane. Believing it was only a matter of time before they themselves were killed, the men started to develop classic stress symptoms: sleep problems, generalized anxiety, colds and flu, fuzzy thinking, short tempers. The expectation of doom effectively disabled a large number of airmen. Then the military leadership had a brilliant idea. They decided to limit the pilots' tour of duty to forty missions. At forty missions, they would be relocated to a safer theater of operations. If a pilot had already done ten missions, he only had thirty to go. If he had done fifteen, he only had twenty-five to go. And so on.

Prior to this decision, the airmen were convinced that it was only a matter of time before their number was up. Sooner or later, they thought, I won't come back. Now, they had hope. When their number was up, they got to go home! The new rule changed their entire perspective, their entire appraisal of danger. When hope was introduced into the equation, pilots regained their function. They still faced dangerous missions, but they were able to finish their tours of duty. Their symptoms of stress disappeared like magic.

From this story I developed the idea of manipulating hope to understand how optimism and pessimism affect the brain. The result was a large-scale study that demonstrated the role that hope, fear, and stress play in shaping our lives. Probably the first scientific study of hope, it involved soldiers who, after a year of advanced training, faced a "final exam" that consisted of a fast, arduous march across the desert with full pack and battle gear. This forty-kilometer (twenty-five-mile) march would have tried anyone's abilities, but it was a distance that the soldiers had successfully completed before. All of the men were experienced, well-conditioned, and highly motivated soldiers who had volunteered to join an elite fighting force. Yet the results revealed huge disparities.

The difference in the soldiers' performance was caused by what they were told about the hike before they began!

There were four sets of test groups. Each group consisted of four platoons. Each platoon had ten soldiers, so there were forty soldiers in each test group and one hundred sixty soldiers being tested overall. Each platoon also had two officers who knew what was actually going on. Each test group was given different information about the length of the march. The study manipulated the soldiers' hopes—and fears—about the difficulty of the march. The goal was to determine what, if any, impact their psychological state had on their physical performance.

Here's how we messed with their minds:

- One set of soldiers was not told how far the march would be.
- One set of soldiers, the control group, was correctly told that they were going to march forty kilometers.
- One set of soldiers was told that they were going to march thirty kilometers (eighteen-plus miles)—25 percent shorter than reality.

- One set of soldiers was told that they were going to march sixty kilometers (thirty-seven miles)—50 percent farther than reality.

They were all going to hike forty kilometers, but they had very different expectations as they began!

Who would perform the best: those with no information, those with the correct information, those with initially encouraging information followed by disappointment, or those with initially discouraging information followed by encouragement? Further, would their psychological and physiological states change once they had the correct information?

We kept track of the number of individuals who successfully completed the march versus their initial expectations about it, and we also took subjective and objective measurements of their physical and mental states along the way.

THE IMPACT OF CORRECT INFORMATION

A rest and food stop was scheduled at twenty-nine kilometers, at which point the two groups with the wrong information were to be set straight about the actual length of the march. The soldiers with no information would not be told the correct length until the end.

However, some of the soldiers failed to make it even that far. Fully *one-third* of the soldiers who believed that they were hiking sixty kilometers dropped out after ten kilometers (six miles)—a distance they normally ran before breakfast each day! Besides the weight of their gear, they were also carrying the weight of "sixty kilometers" in their heads. The early drop-out rate foreshadowed the overall order of finish:

- First place went to the control group of soldiers, who were correctly told that they were going to march forty kilometers.
- Second place went to the group with the optimistic belief that they were going to march only thirty kilometers.
- Third place went to the soldiers who had no idea how long the march would be.

- Last place went to the soldiers who pessimistically thought that they would have to march sixty kilometers instead of forty—another grueling four or five hours longer than they would actually have to go.

We might assume that the best information wins, but that is not the case. *What mattered was how closely the anticipated challenge matched the soldiers' actual capabilities.* Remember, all of them had done a march of this distance and difficulty before. The soldiers with the correct information could compare it with a known achievement. They had little doubt about their ability to succeed. The soldiers who thought that they were marching only thirty kilometers had an unpleasant shock when they discovered the truth. On the one hand, they had already completed three-fourths of the march when they learned the truth, and they had covered the full distance before under similar circumstances. On the other hand, some of them were crushed by the bad news and were unable to finish.

The soldiers in the groups with no information and with pessimistic information fared by far the worst. In fact, there was a big performance gap between the top two and bottom two groups. In common parlance, the last two groups psyched themselves out. For those with no information, the "not knowing" began to exact a toll. More and more of them dropped out toward the end. Those of us who have been on long hikes when we are unsure of the distance can relate to the mental stress of these soldiers. We tell ourselves that our destination is "just over the next ridge," and when we get there we discover that the only thing over the next ridge is . . . another ridge. With every intervening ridge, we lose heart . . . and strength.

It was even worse for the "sixty kilometer" teams. The psychological dread at the prospect of such a long march wrecked this last group. Their minds were consumed from the start with worry about whether they could finish. They began to drop out long before the other soldiers.

The disparity in outcomes among the four groups was so significant that we had to argue with the military not to include the results in the records of the soldiers who had failed. After all, we had manipulated them into lousy performance. This in itself was staggering to contemplate. A simple trick of disinformation had demoralized some of the most physically and psychologically fit human beings in the world—soldiers who had already successfully passed numerous other mental and physical challenges during their combat training.

We made detailed video recordings of the soldiers as they received the correct news at the rest stop. A number of the soldiers who learned that they had to press on for another eleven kilometers became visibly distressed. Many of the men—who a few minutes before had been in good spirits—immediately displayed the kind of flat affect that clinicians associate with depression. Some were literally staggered by the news, and a few even had to lie down. Most had been in good physical shape up until this point, but a disproportionate number dropped out in the last relatively short stretch.

The reaction of the "60K guys" could not have been more dramatically different. It was like watching a fast-motion video of desert flowers blooming after a rain. Upon learning that they had only eleven kilometers to go instead of thirty-one, the soldiers became animated and excited. They exchanged celebratory high-fives. *All of the men in this group who had gotten this far were able to finish.*

The dramatic impact of a shift from negative to positive information is further demonstrated by a nice, unplanned deviation on the study. One of the platoons in the 60K group reached a point at which the soldiers complained vociferously that they could not carry on. It was still fairly early. This commander said to his team: "All of those who want to give up, take one step forward." Practically everybody did. This officer decided to tell his soldiers the truth. "You've seen the crazy psychologist running around here? Well, he's doing an experiment. The march is only 40K, but you weren't supposed to know. All of those who now want to go on, please rejoin the ranks." All of the soldiers did, *and all of them* finished the march. Some of them even ran at the end! By providing good information, the officer saved the day. Without it, he would have been marching by himself.

We took blood samples from the four groups to see how the experience affected each group's stress hormones. Our tests revealed dramatic differences. The soldiers who got bad news at the rest stop (that they would have to carry on longer than they thought) showed sudden spikes in the body's stress hormones—cortisol, epinephrine, and norepinephrine. The soldiers who never knew the actual length of the march were asked at the end to estimate its length. The levels of stress hormones in their blood corresponded to the length *they thought* it was, not the length it *actually* was. Stress hormones do not dissipate fast enough for us to determine whether they dropped for the "60K guys" once they knew the truth. Because the physical exertion was the same for all groups that finished, our blood samplings showed conclusively that the level of stress hormones varied because of psychological, not physical, stress.

We must wonder: All of these soldiers had a proven ability to meet this stern test. Why didn't they all march *at least* the forty kilometers that they had done before? If they all had the resources to achieve the goal, why didn't they? The answer is that the brain does not want the body to expend its resources unless we have a reasonable chance of success. Our physical strength is not accessible to us if the brain does not believe in the outcome, because the worst possible thing for humans to do is to expend all of our resources and *fail*. If we do not believe we can make it, we will not get the resources we need to make it. The moment we believe, the gates are opened, and a flood of energy is unleashed. Both hope and despair are self-fulfilling prophecies.

THROWING COLD WATER ON MORALE

Our project with the soldiers inspired another diabolical test of mind-body interaction. This one involved buckets of cold water. Subjects were required to plunge one of their arms into water that was just a few degrees above freezing. Though not dangerous, the procedure was exceedingly painful. We knew from earlier experiments that most people can keep their arms in the cold water for four minutes. The groups were divided similarly to the soldiers from our earlier experiment:

- One group was told to keep their arms in the cold water for as long as the testers told them to (no information was given as to duration).
- One group was told to keep their arms in the water for four minutes and they could watch the clock (correct information was given).
- One group was told to keep their arms in the water for two minutes. At two minutes they were told, sorry, we meant four (initially encouraging information was given, followed with subsequent disappointment).
- One group was told the test would last for six minutes when in actuality it would last only four minutes (initial discouraging information was given, followed with subsequent encouragement).

After two minutes, the two-minute people and the six-minute people were given the correction information. The people with no information were never told the correct duration. Test results mirrored those of the soldiers on the march. People who had the correct information succeeded most often. People with initially optimistic information did next best, though more of them fell out after they learned the discouraging truth. People with no information fared third best, as their nagging uncertainty had a cumulative negative effect. People who had pessimistic information did the worst, as their dread overwhelmed them—though more of them rebounded once they had the correct information.

We were not done, however. Next, we fooled with the clock. Subjects were told that the test was four minutes, but the actual elapsed time was as short as three minutes or as long as six. If they thought they could do it, they did it. Since then, other researchers have confirmed these outcomes in a variety of settings with people from a number of different backgrounds. They all show that the most important element of success is mental, not physical, strength.

If we can see light at the end of the tunnel, we can handle much more stress than if we see only darkness.

HOPE AS A HEALING AGENT

The impact of a person's mental state is profound. Hope itself counts as an important healing agent. In one medical study, a psychologist conducted a full clinical interview with patients before they had surgery for a hernia. The interview included an evaluation of the person's level of hopefulness. The psychologist found that the patient's recovery time in the hospital was based on their hope index. The more hopeful the patient, the faster and better the healing. A positive connection between hope and healing is supported by a variety of studies. For example, psychologist Barbara L. Frederickson, a MacArthur Award winner at the University of Michigan, found that contentment and joy speed recovery from cardiovascular problems; and a Duke University study showed that heart patients with positive emotions had 20 percent higher long-term survivability rates than those with negative emotions.

Snowdon's analysis of the youthful autobiographies of the nuns he studied also revealed a strong relationship between positive emotions and longevity. Nuns whose essays showed the fewest positive emotions had twice the risk of death at every age versus nuns whose essays showed the most positive emotions. Overall, nuns who were positive in their youth lived on average almost seven years longer than nuns who were pessimistic—in living conditions that were largely identical.

We have all heard stories of the terminal cancer patient who has a few weeks to live, yet against all odds survives another six months to see the birth of a grandchild, dying immediately afterward. Incidents like this turn out to be more than just anecdotal. Several different studies, involving millions of people over several decades, show that terminally ill people repeatedly find a way to live long enough to reach major life milestones such as Thanksgiving, Christmas, and New Year's. Deaths dip just before such milestones and spike just afterward. This "anniversary effect" was documented on January 1, 2000. People made it to the "dawning of the new millennium" and died immediately after. The effect happens every year for the Super Bowl, too. People want to see the big game and enjoy the spectacle! They stick around just long enough to see the final score. The researchers Mitsuru Shimizu and Bret Pelham found that people tend to die on or just after their birthday rather than just before, while the researcher David Phillips concluded that American men tend to die just *before* their birthdays and American women just *after*. Achievement-focused males may dread the "stock-taking" of a birthday, Phillips explains, while socially focused females may look forward to the attention.

Phillips also detected the anniversary effect among Chinese people for the Harvest Moon Festival and among Jewish people for Passover. These studies are significant because the populations surveyed are distinct from the general U.S. population and from each other and because these holidays move around on the calendar. Their impact is completely distinct from seasonal causes of death such as higher levels of serious illness in the winter. (Such seasonal impacts were factored out of the other studies, too, but here the results are especially striking.) For example, elderly Chinese women are the focus of the Harvest Moon Festival, and the dip-and-spike in deaths occurs for them but not for elderly Chinese men or for younger Chinese women.

There is also the folkloric story of elderly U.S. Civil War veterans who made it to a major reunion and then died in inordinate numbers shortly afterward—some of them as they returned home. Handed down through the years, this account could very well be scientifically correct. The most famous anniversary effect involves American presidents. Thomas Jefferson and John Adams both died on July 4, 1826, on the fiftieth anniversary of the signing of the American Declaration of Independence, and James Monroe died five years later on the same date. Three of the five American presidents who were Founding Fathers died on this most special date in the country's history. Somehow people hold on when it means something to them.

Science seems to support the idea that the will to live can carry our failing bodies forward for at least a short time so that we can make a "ceremonial finish line"—a life event that is important to us. Of course, we probably also tend to pay better attention to our medical regimen at such times and receive greater care from family and friends who also want us to live to see the significant event. However, the most likely explanation is that our positive feelings help rally our biology one last time. The anniversary effect is the ultimate evidence that a positive attitude can help us cope with any disease, whether moderately severe or potentially fatal.

Hope also explains the placebo effect, which simply put is that almost any treatment can create a positive effect, even if the treatment is medically neutral. We usually hear of a placebo—an inert substance or sham treatment given to a certain set of patients—being used as a control to determine whether actual medicines or treatments really work. By definition, placebos should have no effect, but study after study shows that they do. Many patients on placebos improve more than untreated patients do, and sometimes they improve as much as patients who are on real treatments. The placebo effect can be so powerful that the makers of Prozac, Paxil, and Zoloft had to run numerous trials to obtain results showing that their drugs worked better than placebos at alleviating depression. The placebo effect occurs for pain, fever, and the immune response, all of which we know can be affected by the conscious mind. The "expectancy effect" appears to be related to the release of dopamine and endorphins, the brain's pleasure and reward chemicals.

All manner of things can activate the placebo effect, ranging from the size and color of the pill that's administered to the attentiveness of the physician to the sophistication of the supposed treatment. When patients perceive that they're receiving complex procedures and expensive pills, they will improve more than if they think that they're receiving simple treatments and cheap pills. People believe that new and costly medicine *must* work better, so they improve.

The healing effect of positive expectations and a positive attitude may explain the benefit of prayer on people who are sick and injured. Many studies have indicated a positive relationship between prayer and recovery. If a patient *believes* that prayers (either their own or those done on their behalf) will lead to a desirable outcome, the brain will likely direct the body to invest more in the healing process. Jeff Levin, an epidemiologist and adjunct professor of psychiatry and behavioral sciences at the Duke University School of Medicine, has reviewed thousands of studies on the relationship between spirituality, health, and healing. Beyond the healthy lifestyles encouraged by most religions and the physical and emotional care often provided by these communities, Levin has identified many studies (he cites about fifty that have been well done) that indicate that faith and prayer help in healing and recovery. They create hope and optimism, the very attitudes that have a self-soothing impact on the immune system and that help rally the body's resources under trying circumstances.

It is not all "Don't worry, be happy." A positive outlook does not guarantee positive results. It only helps. There is a difference between statistics and specifics. The studies say only that across a population, spiritual people live longer and heal better than non-spiritual people. No one can predict what will happen to one particular person. If, for example, a disease has a 25 percent survivability rate, and prayer improves that by 20 percent, then the overall survival rate rises to 30 percent. But *seventy* out of a hundred patients will *still succumb* to the disease. We cannot predict which extra five will survive.

USING PERCEPTION TO HELP TREATMENT

As we have seen, the brain doles out physiological energy based on its perception of whether its efforts will be useful. This knowledge can be put to good use by doctors who are attempting to lead their patients through difficult regimens of care. For example, it is common in cancer treatments for people to require multiple sessions of difficult chemotherapy. If the doctor tells the patient that she needs ten sessions, and she feels wretched after four, she might abandon treatment. Like the marching soldiers, she cannot perceive herself successfully completing six more sessions. If, however, the doctor initially suggests that six treatments will likely do, and the patient feels poorly after four, she will most likely persevere. Two more treatments will probably not seem impossible. After the initial six, the doctor can then tell the patient that the results are so encouraging that he wants to do two more. At eight, he can say the same thing. Eventually, the patient will reach the preferred ten treatments.

This is not to advocate dishonesty with patients. Rather, the suggestion is for physicians to consider the mental component as part of their fundamental treatment strategy, overcoming the brain's unwillingness to release the body's healing powers in the face of seemingly insurmountable obstacles. If many patients struggle to complete a certain regimen, physicians may obtain better results if they break the treatment into shorter, more bearable segments and evaluate the results sooner. If they are encouraging, they can add more segments. This approach gives the mind a winnable goal, encouraging the body to free up its many positive resources, which will help patients undergo the difficult medical trials that could extend their lives.

In any situation the question comes down to manageability. If it is unlikely that a person can achieve a major goal, it is best to break it into mini-goals. Let's assume that we have a problem child in school. Normally, we would reward the child for each day of good manners. However, a child who currently misbehaves a dozen times a day is unlikely to be able to go eight or nine hours without doing something wrong. So we start with a shorter period as the objective, say two hours. When the child goes two hours without any misbehavior, we reward success. Then we gradually extend this period until the child can go the entire day without being naughty. A series of small wins leads to a major victory.

BEING HELPLESS IS NOT THE SAME AS BEING HOPELESS

One final thought involves the difference between helplessness and hopelessness. Years ago, Martin Seligman of the University of Pennsylvania developed the theory that depression is the outcome of learned helplessness, a condition in which a person fails to stop or change a negative situation so often that he or she gives up—even when his or her circumstances change and it is now possible to make things better. The inability to control the situation causes depression, and depression causes the person to stop trying. In his early formulation, Seligman failed to distinguish between helplessness and hopelessness. With their emphasis on active coping, most American people regard the two as equivalent, and in psychological literature the words are often used interchangeably. They are not the same, as a student of mine showed in his doctoral thesis.

A child psychologist, he interviewed a number of children, ranging in age from six to fourteen, about what they would do in a hypothetical stress situation. Imagine yourself going on a trip with friends and family, he told them. You are in the forest and suddenly you realize you are lost. What would you do? The child would say, I will shout for help. He would say, You have shouted, but nobody heard you. The child would say, I will climb up the tree and see how to get out. He would say, You have climbed the tree and could not see a way out. The children he interviewed were wonderful at coming up with ideas about what to do, but he would tell them that each successive idea was inadequate. Finally, they would realize that there was nothing more they could do. They were helpless.

Here the psychologist saw fantastic differences. Some children started to grow anxious and fearful. The psychologist took them gently by the hand, guided them out of the make-believe forest, and calmed them down. Other children, when there was nothing left to try, said, Okay, so I'll just wait for my parents to find me. It's their problem, not mine. These kids were helpless but hopeful. They did not become anxious or afraid of being lost forever. One of the benefits of hope is that it does not imply that we have to solve all of our own problems. Help can come from a family member or a friend, the authorities, a Good Samaritan, God—any outside agent.

The older the children in the study were, the more and more anxious they became toward the end of the interview. Western culture is brainwashing children about the importance of actively controlling their lives. It is good for people to develop a sense of personal responsibility and to take ownership of their problems, but the reality is that much of what happens in life is beyond our control. One of the costs of the strong Western bias for active coping versus emotional coping is that we are lost when we cannot solve our problems.

Seligman eventually changed his theory to account for the many people who did not become hopeless when mired in helpless situations. To come full circle on the main theme of this chapter, it was pessimistic people who tended to fall into hopelessness, while optimistic people did not.

CHOOSING THE RIGHT CANDLE

This series of chapters on stress demonstrates that change and stress are a package deal: Change may be beneficial, but it is also risky. Too much of it in a short period of time becomes stressful. We cannot handle it. Not only do stress hormones physically damage the brain, but a stressed brain bypasses the higher brain functions, settling for whatever solutions the primitive brain deems best for survival. In business and in our personal lives, this rigidity of thought almost guarantees a continuation of the circumstances that originally led to stress. The cycle spirals downward. If we avoid stress entirely, we fall back into the comforts of routine, which has a similar downside of cognitive rigidity and decline.

We need stress in our life if only because we need the stimulus of change. We can use hope, optimism, problem-solving, and emotional support to overcome, or at least alleviate, much of that stress. Enough, at least, to encourage us to embrace the stimulus of change. But some level of stress will always be with us. The question is, how much, at what cost, and for what benefit.

Hans Selye, the pioneer in stress research, was fond of showing everyone a series of photographs of two candles. In the first photo, the candles are the same height and thickness; neither one is lit. They have the same potential. In the second photo, one candle is tucked away in a far corner of the room, barely giving off any light from its lit wick, while the other is next to the window, with lots of air fueling a brilliant flame and wax running down its side. In the third photo, the active candle is finished, used up, while the candle in the corner still slowly burns, only half consumed.

We can have a life that's intense, interesting, and a little bit dangerous. That life will likely be somewhat shorter because of the negative effects of stress. Or we can have a peaceful, long, *dull* life.

Balancing between change and stress on one side and stasis and peace on the other presents to us an important choice. We should all consider a vote for change. The cost to us in terms of stress is more than balanced by an improved quality of life. Change helps us become more cognitively fit and adds spice to what might be an otherwise drab existence.

═══ LESSONS IN BRAINPOWER ═══

- The brain will not let the body expend energy unless it believes that success is possible, because the worst possible thing would be for us to expend all of our resources and *fail*. The moment we believe, the brain unleashes a flood of energy. Both hope and despair are self-fulfilling prophecies.
- Hope itself is an important healing agent. There is a strong connection between recovery from illness and a patient's level of hopefulness and positive thinking. Hope also explains the placebo effect, which occurs when people improve from treatments that have no medical value.
- Doctors should consider the role of positive thinking in designing treatments. The brain is more likely to release the body's healing powers in a series of shorter "winnable" segments than in one long and psychologically daunting regime.
- In general, if it is unlikely that we can achieve a major goal, it is best to break the objective into mini-goals.
- Being helpless is not the same as being hopeless. By maintaining hope, we can persevere until a helpless situation improves.

PART IV

WHAT TO DO

HOW TO BUILD BRAINPOWER FOR A LONG AND HAPPY LIFE

THIRTEEN

Life Is Not Enough to Challenge the Brain

At age seventy-five, Fred has slowed down a lot in the last several years. He has developed balance problems that make him hesitant to go out much. An active man all of his life, he now putters less in the yard and seldom indulges in his beloved hobby of woodworking. His wife, Jane, is seventy-three. She has trouble remembering recent events and activities and has become careless about paying the bills. A spotless housekeeper all her life, she no longer notices dust and clutter and sometimes lets food spoil before cleaning the refrigerator. Fred and Jane's family physician enrolls them in a cognitive training program. In just eight weeks, they make rapid improvement. As their brainpower increases, their physical health improves. They begin to reclaim their lives.

If our lives, like those of our ancestors, were nasty, brutish, and short, then existence itself would be more than enough to keep our brains sharp for the rudimentary survival skills we would need. Our tendency to learn early and well—but then stop learning—would keep us alive, enduring if not prospering. Life in the modern, developed world, however, tends to be long and somewhat uneventful—compared, at least, to what our ancestors suffered, and to what many impoverished people still experience around the world. Fred and Jane learned the hard way that life simply does not challenge our minds enough to keep us healthy.

When I speak about the importance of doing special things to keep the brain in shape, I am often challenged by my audience. "From the moment we wake up until we go to sleep our brains have to attend to complex stimuli," they argue. "We plan many activities—some of them quite complex—we solve many problems, we engage with people, we carry out all kinds of tasks. Isn't our mental exhaustion at the end of the day sufficient proof that we've exercised our brains?"

This line of argument sounds oddly familiar, since it duplicates claims made in the recent past against the need for physical exercise. Not long ago, people tended to say, "Well, I jumped into the elevator and then the car," as if such paltry activities could burn enough calories to keep them fit. It took society many years to realize that the physical exertion required by everyday tasks is far from sufficient. Even a superficial comparison to the activities of people with traditional lifestyles—or our own parents and grandparents—shows that we are not anywhere near physically active enough. In contrast to our hunter-gatherer forebears, we are practically immobilized by creature comforts.

Thank goodness many of us are beginning to say, "Let's take the stairs. Let's go for a walk." People have begun to understand that— particularly as they age—they need to drop unhealthy habits such as smoking and excessive drinking. They know that they need special physical exercise sessions to maintain their cardiovascular health, their muscular strength, and their bone density.

Yet we continue to say, "Well, my life is cognitively challenging," instead of saying, "I need to do more, because most of my mental life is in a rut." Often, the mental exhaustion we feel at the end of the day is related to boredom or stress—psychic frustration—rather than to the heavy lifting of mental exercise. With our overtaxed schedules and busy lives, the last thing most of us want to do is add a regular program specifically designed to stimulate our minds. But then again we used to avoid the gym, too.

TWO WAYS OF THINKING

The main reason for the need of a cognitive regimen is that our brains prefer to take the easier approach to thinking. Whenever we are faced with a problem, we can analyze it to find a new solution or we can refer to similar experiences from our past, evoking an old solution. The first is effortful, time-consuming, and may lead to new insights. The second is quick, easy, and virtually automatic. However, as shown in the early chapters of this book, the convenience of relying on experience may cause us to miss important differences between past experience and the present problem. As a result, the old, familiar solution may be inadequate. Even more critically, reliance on past experience does not offer enough cognitive stimulation today.

The difference between these two ways of thinking can be illustrated in the design of two computer chess programs. The first analyzes the moves of a champion player, assigning different weights to such positional advantages as an open file, a rook in the seventh row, or control of the center of the board. The program mimics the way in which a human might thoughtfully evaluate all of the factors at play before making his or her next move. The second program does nothing more than compile a history of important chess matches and of the moves that led to victory, defeat, or a draw. Based on statistical calculations, the program blindly follows the moves that offer the best chance of victory. It does not need to understand anything more about chess than the moves that are allowed for each piece. If it accumulates enough data, the second program might win more often than the first. And a person who mimicked the latter program's strategy, compiling a similar mental set of known winning moves, might also do well against opponents. But that person would receive virtually none of the cognitive benefits of playing what is for most a challenging and interesting game. Lack of effort would lead him or her straight to cognitive decline.

This example reinforces the pros and cons of both analysis and experience. Undoubtedly, many players learn intuitively by the lat-

ter principle rather than the former, yet the latter also requires practically no thought or effort. Case learning is good when it helps us
make decisions that cannot be easily broken down into logic, but
bad when it turns into a mindless routine.

That the brain by far prefers the automatic mode to the effortful
one feeds directly into our tendency to develop routines. After a few
repetitions, any activity starts to become habitual. Even highly complex intellectual exercises quickly become repetitive. The challenge
decreases. For this reason, everyday life experiences cannot ensure
brain fitness any more than our sedentary lifestyle can assure physical fitness.

Our proposition runs counter to most arguments in favor of experience. In *The Wisdom Paradox*, for instance, neuroscientist Elkhonon Goldberg argues for the value of a senior's lifelong assemblage
of experience. Goldberg has developed an interesting variation on
the standard left-right brain schema. Instead of the right hemisphere
being the creative/non-verbal/musical side and the left hemisphere
being the logical/language side, he proposes that the right side handles the new and the left side handles the familiar. This would explain, for example, why social interactions, which constantly
change, are normally handled on the right side, and why language,
one of the earliest skills we master, is normally found on the left
side. Language becomes part of our left side's "repository of com-
pressed knowledge."

As we age, Goldberg says, our growing experience leads to the
processing of less and less novelty: We see little that is truly new. As
a result, we undergo a "hemispheric shift" in which the majority of
the work in the brain moves from the right side to the left. By ac-
cessing the left side's stored memories through pattern recognition,
we function on cognitive autopilot. Our vault of experience becomes a collection of "wisdom templates" that enable us to replace
the "grinding mental calculations" and intense problem-solving of
youth with the "instantaneous, almost unfairly easy insight" of maturity.

Goldberg's argument is compelling to a point. His notion of a
broad transfer of cognitive control from the right to the left side of
the brain requires more research, but the shift corresponds to what

we would expect for people who begin to rely more and more on experience. While emphasizing the importance of continued stimulation of the mind, Goldberg still seems to think this gradual shift of the mental center of gravity, and reliance on our "wisdom templates," is a good thing—the sine qua non of maturity. However, just as experts are poised on the abyss, about to fall into cognitive decline, so too are overly experienced seniors. *The cognitive decline we see in the elderly is at least partly the direct result of their relying too much on experience.* It is the "grinding mental calculations" that keep us cognitively fit—even if we are not as good at such operations as we were when we were young. Unless we deliberately introduce novelty—learning—to adults with experience, they have no reason to seek out anything new, and their brain begins to atrophy.

TECHNOLOGY HAS ITS DOWNSIDES

Many studies have found a connection between cognitive problems and the number of hours that people spend watching television. Children who exceed the two-hour-a-day recommended maximum for TV or video screen time, for instance, are 1.5 to 2.0 times more likely to have attention and behavior problems than other kids. Usually the rationale given for this disturbing statistic is the "pablum" being shown on the "boob tube." Hundreds of TV channels are available for many people, both on their cable boxes and online. A good deal of the shows must be mediocre or worse at any given moment in time. But then the vast majority of books on the market are not exactly great literature, either. In terms of cognitive decline or gain, what makes the difference between a book (good or bad) and a TV show or movie (good or bad) is the amount of work the brain has to do to comprehend each one.

When A. S. Maulucci opens "Sonnet 33" of his collection *100 Love Sonnets* with these words, "Botticelli would have been inspired / by beauty like yours, by your luminous / face, by the look of dawn in your blue eyes, / by your neck hips thighs flowing like a river," we do not *see* the woman or her beauty. We see black marks on a white page. We must recognize the marks as letters that compose words, and then decode the words so that we can comprehend their meaning. Then we must summon our memories of what the women in Botticelli's paintings look like. And we must puzzle over what emotional or mental state constitutes "dawn in your blue eyes" and how a woman's hips and thighs might flow like a river. Reading just a few short lines requires us to sort through our recollections and stimulate our imaginations to conjure up an image of this tantalizing figure. Because all of our experiences differ, each of us will come up with a different image. One person might bring to mind a particular lost love. Another might invoke a fantasy based on a beauty glimpsed in passing. Another might think of a friend whose attractiveness keeps her from being taken seriously.

The reading experience varies from author to author. Ernest Hemingway guides our perceptions by depicting actions so specifically that we are funneled into thinking a certain way about them. Instead of describing the emotions themselves, his approach is to describe "the exact sequence of events" that leads to them. He uses simple words and sentence structures (though not as simple as most people believe) so that our minds become engaged in the situation itself rather than in the writing. William Faulkner and James Joyce, on the other hand, use a complexity of style, structure, and vocabulary to absorb us in another way. We become enmeshed in the rhythm of their writing and the intricacy of their word choices. When reading these authors we are apt to become lost in a symphony of internal sound. Much of our mental energy is absorbed in understanding what they are actually saying and how they are saying it. There are brackets within brackets within brackets, and we have to be on guard not to lose track of a nested statement.

Compare the considerable cognitive effort required for reading a book with that required for television. Rather than imagining a woman with the flush of dawn in her eyes, we turn on the TV, and a beautiful blue-eyed woman appears before us. No assembly required. The mind reacts rather than creates. The cognitive effort is close to zero.

There is also the "cut-away effect" created by commercials; we become invested in a story only to have it interrupted every ten minutes or so for advertising. The brain is so clever that it begins to anticipate these disruptions and cruises along at a shallow level. Children who watch a lot of TV develop shorter attention spans (10 percent shorter for every hour watched per week). We are training these kids and other TV viewers *not* to become too involved in the story. This problem, however, is a result of the structure of most TV programming; it is not inherent in the medium. It is TV's passive nature that causes the primary problem, not the content or the commercial breaks per se.

Visual media can challenge the mind, of course. Movies such as *The Matrix* or *Inception* use visual effects that stimulate thought by challenging our assumptions about reality. And three-dimensional digital presentations can radically improve learning for complex subjects such as chemistry, astronomy, and engineering. They enable us to see the physical results of mathematical and chemical formulas. "The Inner Life of the Cell," an animation of the real structures and processes within the cell, is a good example of how the visual arts can take us to worlds that we cannot otherwise fathom.

For the most part, however, the visual presentation of information is a cognitively cheaper replacement for the more difficult process of reading. Email has replaced the harder work of letter-writing and the stimulation of personal meetings, and texting and tweeting have become simpler forms of email. This electronic brevity insulates us from the more mentally challenging interactions that used to make up most of our workday and leisure time. For all their good, new technologies reduce our overall cognitive effort. GPS, for instance, stimulates the minds of a small number of engineers who develop the products, while causing users to lose spatial awareness because it's easier to follow "George" than to navigate manually. Critical industries such as nuclear power and commercial aviation struggle with the issue of mental alertness and agility for humans overseeing increasingly automated systems. Every technical advance simplifies another bit of cognitive work that we used to do ourselves. Bit by bit, the loss adds up.

BUILDING BRAIN CELLS ONE WORKOUT AT A TIME

If life is not enough to challenge our brains, then what are we to do? Let's start at the gym. As touched upon in Chapter 6, physical exertion causes more blood to flow to the brain, improving its function. And that's not the only benefit our brains get from exercise. It also leads directly to the creation of new brain cells! The relationship between exercise and cell regeneration was first discovered in laboratory rats. Rodents that spent more time in their exercise wheels did better on mazes and other tests than their lazier brethren. When scientists delved deeper, they discovered that exercise led to a doubling or tripling of the number of newborn cells in the hippocampus and other parts of the brain. Exercising animals also showed reduced damage, and faster recovery, from strokes.

Arthur Kramer and his fellow researchers, who had previously confirmed the positive effect of exercise on cognition, later demonstrated how exercise actually changes the brain. In one test, they compared the cognitive skills of physically fit people with those of physically unfit people. In another, they compared the cognitive skills of people who had done aerobic exercise for six months with those who had done only stretching and toning for that same period. In the cognitive tests, subjects had to pick out one object from among other distracting objects, in what is known as a "flanker" problem. Symbols such as > > > > > and > > < > > were flashed across a screen. By pressing a button on the left or on the right, the subject indicated which way the center arrow was pointing. The speed and accuracy of the response indicated how good the subject was at ignoring the distracting symbols on the flank.

The physically fit adults were consistently more efficient in dealing with conflicting flanker cues. The less physically fit had more difficulty with incongruent flanker cues. The group that began practicing aerobics showed significant cognitive improvement, but the "stretch and tone" group showed no improvement over the sedentary group. Physical changes in the brain corresponded with the cognitive results. The aerobic exercisers experienced growth in the attentional areas of the cortex. The people who were physically fit already had larger areas in these regions of the brain. The toners and the sedentary group showed little or no brain growth. The lesson: Exercise grows the brain the way it routinely grows muscles. Studies of laboratory animals show that the increased volume comes from the growth of more blood vessels, increased connections between brain cells, the development of new neurons, the longer life of existing neurons, and greater efficiency in the neurotransmitter system. Kramer et al concluded that even short-term exercise programs can restore at least some age-related losses in brain volume.

As a side note, studies on mice have shown that radiation interferes with the integration of exercise-induced connections (learning), but that continued exercise can lessen and often even reverse these negative effects. Radiation treatment is common for childhood brain cancer, and cognitive deficits are sometimes the result. This indicates that exercise programs may be especially beneficial not only for people with cognitive concerns but also for those who have received radiation therapy—or any other trauma—related to the brain. Lance Armstrong's remarkable recovery from testicular cancer, which had spread into his brain, included grueling months on an exercise bike. That he went on to win multiple Tours de France and has remained healthy may be a testament to the benefits of exercise beyond heart and lung conditioning.

Though it is clear why improved blood flow boosts brain function, it is more of a mystery why exercise itself would lead to the creation of neurons. If we accept the postulate of one writer that only a moving animal requires a brain, we may begin to have an inkling about the interrelationship between our physical and mental development. The brain occupies only 2 percent of our body mass, and yet it uses 20 percent of the body's resting glucose output and 25 percent of its oxygen. (This intense energy use is what requires us to wear a hat in frigid conditions to avoid hypothermia.) For any organism, from the smallest field mouse to a human being, having a brain and its ability to adapt to stimulus must provide many advantages in order to justify these enormous costs. Being able to develop strategies for finding food and a mate is likely one major benefit. Being able to travel long distances, which many animals routinely do, must confer benefits as well—more food, safer reproductive sites, fewer competitors and predators. A brain that grows when physically challenged must improve the odds of survival for any kind of travel, including migrations. Frederick Gage, one of the discoverers of neuronal stem cells in the adult brain, calls the effect of exercise on neurons "anticipatory proliferation"—we form new brain cells in preparation for a new environment. Undergoing physical stress today in a jog down a tree-lined street or on a treadmill in the sanctuary of a fitness club may trigger the same biological response as when we prepared to track and kill game or explore the far horizons.

THE CASE FOR BRAIN EXERCISE

Because there are limits to the variety and challenge implicit in modern life—and limits to what most of us can afford in terms of time or money to achieve this variety—it makes sense for us to make specific investments in cognitive training, just as we do in physical training. When it comes to brain teasers, crossword puzzles, Sudoku, math and word puzzles, and other such brain fodder, most people do *not* understand the speed with which they hit diminishing returns. The brain's adaptability enables it to quickly figure out the underlying logic and patterns of word and math games and mental puzzles. The challenge of these exercises falls off rapidly. Think back to Mike Merzenich's study about how the brain first responds to challenges by expanding connections and then by consolidating them. If we route things from A to B to C to D to E and always end up at F, the brain will eventually go directly from A to F, pruning the other unnecessary connections. In addition, the skills we develop from practicing games do not task us in enough different ways to improve our overall cognitive abilities.

On a recent airplane trip, I had finished my book and was looking for something to occupy the time. I was glad to find a crossword puzzle in the in-flight magazine. It turned out to be too difficult for me, because it was filled with questions related to television shows that I had not seen. I quickly lost interest. On other occasions, easy crosswords have likewise failed to hold my interest. The optimal level of challenge for a crossword is when the puzzle is easy enough to get at least some words on the first pass but too difficult to get all of them. With the puzzle partially solved and a few new letters serving as clues, we can go back and fill in other words we did not know the first time. As we solve more words, we get more clues. Stage by stage, we complete the puzzle. However, with a crossword, Sudoku, or any similar game, it is a matter of luck as to whether the puzzle proves to be the right level of difficulty.

The computer turns out to have significant advantages in terms of cognitive training. It is an irony that the computer—a device that is very, very dumb, but very, very fast—can help produce a program of mental exercises that will help the much more clever human brain stay in shape. One of the reasons is that a computer is capable of monitoring every task a person does on it. It can measure the time it takes for a person to respond to a question down to the millisecond. It can measure resolution to the level of a single pixel, so that it can precisely determine the user's actions in terms of spatial awareness. This instant and constant measuring allows for the creation of adaptive software. While a person is working on one test or puzzle, the computer can start determining what the next one should be. The optimal level, of course, differs for each person, so individualized training is important.

A number of computerized cognitive training programs exist, including those produced by my own company. Some of these programs are very good, and some of them are not. Individuals can do a number of things to ensure that a cognitive training program will have value for them. First and foremost, they can research the credentials of the company's founders and its senior executives. The important personnel should have educational backgrounds in pertinent fields and have experience at universities or other relevant organizations. It's a plus if they have published research in independent journals.

Next, consumers should take a good look at the research behind the company's products. The BBC, which has done a number of reports on the brain and on brain-training software, has identified five major requirements in evaluating the science behind cognitive training software. They are worth a mention here:

Peer review. Consumers should look beyond a company's promotional materials and anecdotal user testimonials and instead seek out peer-reviewed articles in independent publications. Studies about a company's methodology and tests should be done by independent scholars, and the conclusions should be reviewed by other independent researchers. The same entity promoting the product cannot be the one validating it.

Brain imaging. Researchers should be able to predict which areas of the brain will be affected by the training, and brain scans—comparing scans of an individual's brain from before and after the training program—should validate these predictions. The amount of learning that occurs must be validated by separate tests. A brain scan is a tool for research, not an end in itself.

Control groups. A legitimate study must compare results from the test group with results from control groups. Otherwise, there is no way to tell whether it was the brain-training program that provided the benefit or whether it was the result of *any* other uses of the brain.

A major study carried out by the BBC discovered that one six-week brain training program led to no more improvement in cognitive fitness than did trolling for information on the Internet. The subjects' brains quickly adapted to the repetitive nature of the program's games, which did not increase in difficulty. The value of the training soon evaporated. Serious training software goes far beyond this.

Benchmark. A benchmark for cognitive fitness software is a cognitive test taken before and after the training program to determine how much performance has improved through training. A cognitive benchmark needs to challenge the brain differently from the training software. Some manufacturers use benchmark tests that are very nearly identical to the tests given during training. In such a case, all that is being demonstrated is that practice on one set of mental tasks leads to an unsurprising improvement on similar tasks. The purpose of cognitive fitness software is that we can transfer our cognitive gains to many different mental tasks.

Individuality. Consumers should pick a program that is likely to produce good results for someone whose profile is similar to theirs. For example, a program designed for seniors might focus on mental skills such as memory, which will be helpful for them, but less so for young people. Some programs provide a standard set of tests, regardless of the cognitive ability of the test-taker. Others are capable of producing only a little variety. If the program is too easy, the subject will get bored; if it's too hard, he or she will become discouraged.

A brain-training program should begin with a series of exercises that enables the software to gauge the user's ability level. Based on this initial round of tests, he or she should be presented with challenging but not impossible tasks. As the user gets better—and the brain becomes efficient (lazy)—the program should escalate in difficulty just enough to keep the person engaged. This process should continue for as long as the person uses the program.

A cognitive training program that has all of the qualities discussed above can improve the mental function of a variety of people. The improvements often result from an increase in our working memory, which processes new stimuli. Most of us can commit seven or eight single items to memory at a time before the information begins to decay. These items can be such mundane things as a phone number or the name of a person who was just introduced to us. The effective span of our working memory affects everything we do.

A study done by the University of Haifa in Israel is illustrative. Researchers sought to determine whether brain-training software could improve the reading skills of adult dyslexics. Dyslexia is a learning disability in which the brain has difficulty decoding graphic symbols such as letters and words. An electric signal is triggered in the frontal lobes whenever the brain notices a mistake. This "error wave" presumably begins the process of correction. In dyslexics, the error wave is much smaller than in regular readers, implying a reduced ability either to sense or correct mistakes. The Haifa researchers predicted that cognitive training would reduce dyslexics' reading mistakes by increasing their working memory and thus their brains' ability to detect and correct errors. The change would be indicated by an increase in the size of the error wave and validated by demonstrated improvements in reading.

Dyslexic subjects and a control group of normal readers, all of whom were Haifa University students, were tested three times for working memory and reading skills: at the beginning of the study, after six of weeks of cognitive training, and after six months. The training—twenty minutes a day, for four days a week—increased the size of the error wave by nearly 25 percent in dyslexic subjects, almost to the size found in normal readers. More important, the larger error wave corresponded both with better working memory and an improvement in reading. The "digit span" of the dyslexic students, for instance, increased by one item from the first test to the third, from 9.8 to 10.8. Their reading skills increased significantly, by an average of nearly 15 percent. The control group of normal readers also improved, though not as much as the dyslexics. Both normal readers and dyslexics retained most of their gains after six months, with normal readers retaining slightly more. The three sets of benchmark tests were of a totally different nature than the cognitive training program. (The university used one of my company's products as the training software, but we were not otherwise involved.) The study results were accepted for publication in a peer-reviewed journal.

Another fascinating example comes to us from the Albert Einstein School of Medicine in New York. Falling is a major danger for the elderly, often leading to broken hips or other injuries that can lead to serious physical decline and even death. The Einstein School researched possible ways to improve the walking skills of elderly patients, reducing their risk of falling. The primary test involved having the patients think and talk as they walked. For example, they might be asked to recite aloud every other letter of the alphabet (A, C, E, . . .). The patients wore sensors that enabled the scientists to measure how well they walked as they carried out the assignment.

THE IMPACT OF HARD COGNITIVE WORK

By improving attention, perception, and short-term memory, cognitive training should create general improvement in mental function, beyond the tasks that are used in the exercises themselves. Significant results have been obtained from a variety of scientifically valid brain-training regimens.

- As previously mentioned, children with learning disabilities caused by the slow processing of sounds in the brain ended up with normal or better language scores after an eight- to twelve-week cognitive training program. They did much better than a control group and retained the gains after a six-week retest. A follow-up study involving 500 children with learning disabilities showed an average improvement of 1.8 years in language development after six weeks of training.
- Older adults who underwent annual cognitive training over a five-year period declined less in the functions of daily life than others in their cohort who did not undergo training.
- After rigorous preparation for their board exams, medical students were found to have significant structural brain changes related to improved memory.
- College students randomly selected for three months of training in the art of juggling had increases in brain volume in the areas related to motor skills. A three-month follow-up showed that they retained most of the gains after juggling lessons stopped.

In between walking tests, some patients underwent cognitive training. The cognitive drills consisted of twenty-minute sessions three times a week for eight weeks, a total of eight hours of work. Patients who did cognitive training walked better both *without* talking and *while* talking than those who did not take training. The improvement was still visible two months after the end of training. The software used for training had nothing to do with gait. It had to do with improving attention and memory. The elderly patients could walk and talk—without falling—because cognitive training helped them develop spare cognitive capacity.

MASTERY BRINGS EXCITEMENT

My sister, who is four years older than I am, had never touched a personal computer. It was her decision. She simply did not believe that PCs were for our generation. Seeing this as a terrible waste, our family tried to change her mind. Here was an intelligent, healthy woman who was denying herself access to so many things—emails and photos relating to her grandchildren, easy communication with distant friends and relatives, and all of the other benefits of being instantly in touch with people around the world.

Fortunately, she became worried about her memory. When my company began developing cognitive-training programs, she kept asking me, "When will you have the brain software?" Finally it was ready, and we installed it on her husband's computer. I didn't chaperone her. I told her that the program would guide her through the steps. Of course, she didn't know how to use a mouse. Fortunately, the brain is very good at learning and retaining motor skills, which is why we never forget how to ride a bike. It took her about forty-five minutes to figure out the mouse, and then she was off and running with the software.

Mastering the computer was significant in itself, independent of the brain-training program. She was excited by her ability to learn something new and complicated. Psychologically, she underwent a transformation. She was no longer an outsider to the world of computers and the Web. She was "with it" in regards to technology. Her new confidence was bolstered when she mastered still other PC skills and started developing electronic relationships.

I have seen this kind of positive response in other seniors. Many of the elderly have a general sense that everything is getting harder. They feel that they are in the grips of an unstoppable physical and mental decline. Unsurprisingly, their morale suffers. Depression may set in. (This is the downward spiral that Fred and Jane, the aging couple from the beginning of the chapter, faced in their lives.) Then they master a new challenge—the Internet or a musical instrument or a brain-training program. Exercises that were difficult yesterday become easier to do today. Seniors realize that life is far from over; progress is possible. The lesson of the soldiers' arduous march through the desert is that when we believe we have a chance to win, the brain commits its resources to winning. The initial gains from brain training or other effortful activities convince the mind that bigger victories are possible. This type of positive reinforcement occurs quickly with computerized training because the feedback is immediate and positive.

Brain training, then, has both a specific effect on cognitive vitality and a non-specific effect on our overall psyche. It improves our underlying cognitive skills, which then improve all of the mental activities based on these skills. The proof of good cognitive training is not an improvement on the benchmark test or in the training program itself. The proof is in how much of the benefit carries over into regular life. If dyslexics improved on the benchmark but not in regular reading, or if the elderly got faster in their cognitive tests but still suffered from falls, what would be the point? The dyslexics were not trained to read, but they could read better. The elderly did not receive gait training, but they could walk better. These are the kinds of outcomes, based on improvements in the underlying cognitive skills of attention, perception, and short-term memory, that matter.

In addition, the morale boost that older people get when they master something new—it's magic. I make the claim, only partly in jest, that if brain-training programs have no positive impact beyond giving seniors a sense of accomplishment, that's probably good enough! Even simple games can give people a confidence boost because they do get better with practice. We know when a task is too easy, so we get the most psychic reinforcement when we master a difficult task. The optimal level of challenge is good for both specific and non-specific effects. We learn that we have to expend effort to experience pleasure. That, in turn, motivates us to try more.

══ LESSONS IN BRAINPOWER ══

- Just as we need regular exercise for our bodies, we need regular exercise for our brains. Daily life does not provide enough stimulation or mental variety to keep the brain at its mental peak.
- In some respects, technology makes life too easy for us. With steadily declining cognitive effort, we must find offsetting ways to stimulate the brain.
- Good cognitive training programs provide the same "toning" benefits to the mind that good exercise programs provide to the body. Cognitive fitness programs should meet rigorous standards, including individualization and a steady increase in difficulty as the user improves.
- The goal of cognitive training is not to improve in speed or results on computer tests or games but to improve our actual functioning in the real world.

FOURTEEN

Occupational Agility

After a comfortable forty-year career in academia as a psychology professor, I did what any rational sixty-five-year-old would do upon retirement. I took some of my life savings and started a new company in an untried field. If that wasn't enough, a few years later I ran for and won a seat in my country's parliament. What doesn't kill us makes us . . . more cognitively fit?

Though my choices were voluntary, many people in today's world find that they have to switch jobs—and even fields—much more often than was the case in the past. For most of their working years, Baby Boomers could count on large companies to provide long-term if not lifetime employment. Yet by the time they turned forty-four, most of them had worked in more than eleven different jobs or fields. The pace of change has undoubtedly accelerated in the last decade as businesses downsized, outsourced, or regularly reorganized, often leaving employees out of jobs. Lower-skill jobs continue to move to lower-cost countries. To stay competitive, companies must continually innovate. A valid job description for today may be obsolete tomorrow. As a result, workers who stay with a company must be willing and able to adapt to ever-changing circumstances at work. This new reality implies that management-employee relations need to shift from adversarial to cooperative, but there is little indication that such a shift in mind-set is occurring broadly on either side.

In response to the grim realities of today's economy, employees now feel much less loyalty to their employers than previous generations did. Workers are apt to jump to a new position—or start their own businesses—before being pushed. This attitude adds to the instability because employers tend to lose their most skilled employees.

Whether within a company or between companies, whether forced or voluntary, change is something for which most people are unprepared. But if an individual has only one narrow set of skills, tailored to a particular profession, technological or economic disruptions can be disastrous. This is also true in nature. A species that is too snugly adapted to a single environment can be wiped out by a radical change. Luckily, evolution provides species with mechanisms to deal with such upheavals. Two variations of the Arizona pocket mouse live close to each other in the Southwest American desert. They come from the same stock, a mouse that naturally produces offspring of variable color. The light pocket mouse lives on the light-colored desert sand, and the dark pocket mouse lives on dark-colored lava. The populations have become distinct over the years because mice that blended in with their respective backgrounds lived long enough to reproduce. The ones that did not blend in got picked off by predators. Modest color variability enables the mouse to exist in either environment.

Most species have enough variations encoded in their genes to survive at least some environmental changes. A striking example involves lizards that were moved by biologists from one island in the Adriatic Sea to another, where their primary food source changed from insects to vegetation. Within thirty-six years, new generations of the transplanted lizards developed more powerful jaws for chewing plants and new structures in their digestive tracts—cecal valves—which improved their digestion of plant material. Cecal valves, which occur in less than 1 percent of all scaled reptiles, had never been found in this species before.

In today's unforgiving work environment, many people find themselves as displaced as the Adriatic lizards. A single lifespan is too short to bring genetic variability into play, but humanity's greatest inherited trait is our natural adaptability to new environments. We may be the only species that lives in every clime, and it's because we don't have to physically adapt. We adapt with our tools, ingenuity, and organizational ability. Workers must use these innate human qualities to cultivate the skills to protect themselves from economic unpredictability. Our ability to successfully adjust to change is based on how diverse our knowledge and abilities are.

Changing careers is one of the most difficult endeavors that any of us can undertake, but it can also be the most rewarding. Not just personally or financially but also cognitively. What I learned by stepping outside the traditional role of an academic was how differently people think in different professions.

A scholar's frame of reference is defined by the desire to study interesting problems and to develop answers that are provably correct. A scholar thinks, "Give me a problem, give me some money, give me ten years, and I will attempt to find an answer that is one hundred percent correct." Often the "problem" being studied is abstract and theoretical. A businessperson thinks in terms of what can be achieved immediately under budget constraints. Businesspeople forego the need to be scientifically accurate and to understand all conceivable ramifications in order to find a practical solution to a real problem. Their thinking is usually concrete and directly applicable to daily life. Professors consider a topic for research primarily on the basis of what interests them the most. A businessperson must figure out what interests others the most—and what they're willing to pay for it. This difference is why scientists primarily do basic research and businesses focus on applied research.

Politics is another matter entirely. Politicians need to keep their constituents and their parties happy and to seek solutions that will be satisfactory to as many people as possible (most of whom have contradictory interests). Such an approach means very few solutions are "correct"—only workable. At times, even good solutions are rejected because they work against the short-term interests of the very parties that would benefit! On both the left and the right, we see politicians reject compromise because an improvement in the situation would give them less to complain about. Compared to the analytic skills required in other professions, politics requires emotional intelligence, "street smarts," and an inordinate amount of patience.

In considering the differences between academia, business, and politics, it struck me that succeeding in these different professions was not just a matter of learning new and different tasks and a new culture, which are themselves mentally stimulating. It was also a matter of developing a different mental framework for each one. Of introducing variety not just to *what* we think but *how* we think. In pondering this matter and talking it over with colleagues, I came up with at least seven different modes of thought. They are:

1. Scientific. Defines reality as that which can be measured. Accepts as fact only what can be derived by a specific progression of reason, reproducible experiments, or an overwhelming compilation of supporting evidence. Solves complex questions by breaking them down into increasingly simple components until the individual components can be solved. Emphasizes precision, logic, and the controlling of variables so that one item can be measured at a time. Develops fundamental explanatory principles that can be expressed formally (e.g., equations).

2. Legal. Interprets reality according to founding principles and (usually) a body of law that accumulates over time. Emphasizes precedent and adherence to tradition. Legal thinking and strategy vary by country because of underlying cultural differences. English and American law begins with the rights of individual citizens. The Napoleonic Code, which underlies many European and some Arabic systems, begins with the power of the state. The essence of legal thinking is to find the central issue in a case that relates to a firmly established legal principle and build an argument from there. Concerned with details, precedents, related rulings, and formal process.

3. Literary. Creates reality through images, words, and the rhythm of language. Enables people to experience the lives of others through exposure to the full spectrum of human expe-

rience. Delves into the psyche of people; raises questions of emotional intelligence and empathy.

4. Historical/anthropological. This involves analyzing situations by exploring their antecedents. It requires an understanding of the evolving story of humankind and an application of the lessons of yesterday to today's cultural and political contexts. Like the literary mode of thinking, historical shares an interest in underlying motives. Whereas literary emphasizes individual motivation, historical emphasizes the context of an action, i.e., the background circumstances such as cultural or political clashes, large migrations, food shortages, and the like. Historical thinking can mean changing a precedent rather than following it—learning what not to do. As George Santayana said, "Those who cannot remember history are condemned to repeat it."

5. Business. Making real things work, and work quickly. Determining what offers enough value that people will trade items of corresponding value for it. How solutions can be built, distributed, and marketed efficiently throughout complex systems. How the value received can be translated into still more products. Raises questions of the size of the market and barriers to entry, costs, time to market, competition, etc. Constant weighing of practical trade-offs.

6. Political. "The art of the possible," as the German Chancellor Bismarck once said. Bismarck is also the one who described laws as being like sausage: It's better not to see them being made. Political thinking includes the ability to understand multiple points of view, the art of compromise, and the capacity to perceive opportunities in the large number of constraints, conflicts, and pressures of public engagement. Raises issues of feasibility, anticipated opposition, quid pro quo, short-term versus long-term benefits, common ground, etc.

7. Ethical. This mode of thinking emphasizes moral values in decision making. The question is not whether a course of action is scientifically, politically, or legally correct but whether it is ethically and morally correct. Ethical thinking often runs

parallel to other modes of thought (though it is sometimes in conflict with them). Puts the question of values above all other considerations.

We might also ask to what degree a problem requires in-depth knowledge and prior experience, a perspective that would apply to all seven categories.

Current research seeks to broaden the notion of intelligence from the narrow conception measured by IQ. Howard Gardner, for example, has proposed nine different kinds of intelligence that are part of humanity's inherited cognitive arsenal. Kinesthetic intelligence is one of Gardner's categories: how our minds understand the world through the physical manipulation of objects. Some people have a knack for three-dimensional and mechanical designs and tasks that others lack. Artists, for instance, are people who perceive reality and express their thoughts and emotions in various physical ways. Kinesthetic differences can be seen as early as childhood; some children appear to learn better through physical interaction than through abstract thought. As an extreme example, autistics, who have trouble comprehending social interactions, often benefit from hands-on learning. Some educators seek to map educational approaches to a child's perceived natural learning style, though most children learn best by being engaged through several different approaches (sight, sound, touch) rather than through just one. Learning is strongest when it is reinforced in multiple ways.

There may be some overlap between Gardner's categories of intelligence and the seven modes of thought outlined earlier. For example, his "musical intelligence" would be a combination of the literary and mathematical modes. The difference is that a particular kind of intelligence is part of an individual's inherited abilities, while our seven modes of thought are cognitive skills that can be enhanced through exposure and application. The musical talent of Amadeus Mozart, the mathematical talent of Isaac Newton, and the literary talent of Iris Murdoch are the result of the inherent way the brains of these artists worked. It's a *kind* of intelligence. Through effort, the rest of us can develop passable skills at music, math, and writing. Learning the seven different modes of thought will benefit us cognitively, even if we have no native genius—no special kind of intelligence—that makes us a master of this realm.

We can think of these modes as seven different people who, when confronted with the same issue, all ask very different questions about it. The most difficult matters require the use of several different mental perspectives before the best solution presents itself. Consider the advantage of having seven different thinkers inside our head! For this reason, exposure to multiple modes of thought should be part of the education of all young people.

IN PRAISE OF GENERALISTS

This discussion leads us to the classical distinction between specialists and generalists. Our argument is for generalists. If we know a lot about a little and have to change professions, we will probably not be prepared for new work. One reason is that specialists exercise their brains deeply in only one way. Another reason is that, as the world becomes more complex, fewer and fewer answers can be found within the walls of a single discipline. The distinctions between traditional disciplines are becoming very blurry and arbitrary.

We have learned so much about every field that most new questions fall across the borders of two or three disciplines. Quantum theory engages the previously separate fields of chemistry and physics, calling on the expertise of scientists studying everything from the smallest particles to the largest structures in the universe. Practical research, too, has also begun to involve multiple disciplines. The United States has commissioned three energy innovation hubs—focused, respectively, on nuclear energy, solar energy, and energy conservation—to bring together scientists and engineers from different fields in order to stoke creativity. IEEE, the worldwide association of engineers, has convened a special multidisciplinary smart-grid task force to generate new solutions to power distribution and management. Scientists from different fields teamed up at UCLA to figure out how to capture the image of the atomic structure of the adenovirus, a structure smaller than the wavelength of light and thus invisible by most methods. Their success may enable the use of this virus to target medication for gene therapy and cancer. Toyota revolutionized automobile manufacturing by using "obeya"—the word means "big room"—to put designers, engineers, and production staff in a single place.

In terms of cognition, a multidisciplinary approach changes not only the outcome but also *how we think*. A good example involves four New Jersey hospitals, which were examined for how they treated congestive heart problems. There were two wealthy hospitals, one with good results and one with poor results, and two financially strapped hospitals, one with good results and one with poor results.

The hospitals that were struggling were organized in traditional medical fashion. Most of the doctors were independent professionals who made little effort to integrate their individual craft with the larger organization. The culture was a traditional status system in which doctors' orders were followed without question. The hospitals that provided good, cost-effective health outcomes did so through a collaborative approach. Multidisciplinary teams of doctors and nurses did rounds to observe patients, and multidisciplinary committees reviewed and standardized the quality of care. These hospitals empowered nurses—the people who typically spend the most time with patients—as coordinators. They also systematically uncovered and fixed problems. One team improved inventory management, an aspect of cost control that no group within the hospital, certainly not the doctors, would ever have focused on separately.

Many of the difficulties of the struggling hospitals stemmed from cognitive rigidity, reinforced by years of experience (doing the same things the same way) and a culture that celebrated both status and the status quo. Most of the decision makers were specialists. No one was trained in the concept of tackling issues from multiple directions. No one understood that solving problems at the global level, collaboratively, would improve the patients' experience and make their own lives easier.

A multidisciplinary approach took everyone out of rigid ways of doing things, inspiring fresh thinking. Doctors, in particular, were forced to deal directly with the real problems trailing in their wake; they could not walk away from confusing or contradictory treatment orders. Standardized procedures and the adoption of digital technology helped to further reduce errors and duplication. But the biggest long-term gains came from the mental shift: a willingness to listen to other healthcare providers, including nurses; and a dawning awareness that runaway costs are as much a symptom of inefficiency in hospitals as they are in any other arena.

The success that hospitals have achieved through collaboration is by no means unusual. The World Health Organization has developed a surgical checklist that emphasizes communication and teamwork in the operating room. The checklist, which has been implemented in more than twenty countries, has reduced surgical deaths by nearly half, from 1.5 percent to 0.8 percent, while dropping the number of surgical complications from 11 to 7 percent. The list was developed on principles espoused by Atul Gawande in *The Checklist Manifesto*. Gawande believes that the complexity of most fields exceeds the ability of even experts to perform consistently and safely. Checklists are not just memory aids. They ensure that everyone involved in a situation speaks up and that problems are approached from multiple points of view, so that the chances of errors are greatly reduced.

It is safe to predict that most future breakthroughs in science and business will occur at the intersection of multiple fields. On the organizational level, the contrast in results is so stark that we can draw a general rule: Every successful complex organization uses a collaborative, multidisciplinary approach. Every failure depends on an inflexible hierarchy. What does all of this mean on the individual level? The growing need for workers to be able to collaborate across disciplines requires a broader, more general education. Only people who have some knowledge of a number of fields can take advantage of all of the opportunities presented by our modern world.

THE LESSON OF THE LIBRARY

I once spent three weeks in the National Library of Medicine to study immunology. I was the first person in each day and the last to leave. This was before the age of electronic files. I spent a fortune on copies. I spent my nights studying at the Bethesda, Maryland, Holiday Inn, with all of the articles spread around the floor of my room.

As a psychologist, I had some medical background. It was very hard to learn a new area with hundreds of new definitions and ideas. As I found my way, though, learning slowly became easier. The technical terms became more familiar; concepts began to sink in. The more important messages started to pop up—they asked to be read. I began to make sense of the field, but it took every iota of my cognitive skills.

The work challenged my brain as nothing had in many years. Like my sister when she finally learned how to use a computer, I gained a confidence boost: We can successfully cross career boundaries and delve into subject matter that is remote from our existing body of knowledge. Studying a new field also enables us to make new connections that we would never have been able to see before. It creates a multidisciplinary team in our own head.

One of the things I learned in my weeks of study was the "lock and key" mechanism by which the body's white blood cells latch onto foreign cells, which is the first step in killing them. For the docking to occur, the shape of the receptor (a protein on the surface of the T-cell) must match the shape of the antigen (a protein on the surface of the invasive cell). But the fit does not have to be precise. It only has to be close—good enough, in other words. Imprecision is a tremendous advantage, as it dramatically reduces the number of keys the body needs to bust the locks of bad cells. Like the earlier example in which the immune system first ignores a harmless mutation, then ignores a similar one that is cancerous, the immune system is again exhibiting a "satisfycing" principle. This "good enough" reaction is analogous to the brain's response when confronted with similar experiences.

The physical forms of convergent evolution have long been recognized. Wings in birds and bats, for example, evolved from separate physical structures under similar evolutionary pressure. But satisfycing is more of a *principle* (an idea) than an identifiable structure (a thing), and it arose separately in both our cognitive and immunological systems! This insight, that evolution provides multiple pathways for similar concepts as well as for similar physical structures, has stayed with me.

Cognitive skills bloom through our involvement in radically different pastimes. My multiple career experiences taught me the value of learning completely different ways of thinking about the world and solving problems. Brainwidth increases because the very nature of the problem to be solved differs radically in various professions. Exposure to multiple disciplines gives us the ability to solve problems more broadly, just as specialists from multiple disciplines can solve complex organizational problems more effectively if they collaborate than if they work in isolation. Different occupations also force us out of cognitive ruts. The ultimate value of the three weeks in the library was not *what* I learned, but *that* I learned.

We will have these broader skills at the ready when we need them—though we can never know when that will be. Just as a diversified investment portfolio protects people from serious downturns in particular market segments, a diversified portfolio of skills provides greater job protection in a difficult economy. People need a broad portfolio of skills to help them adapt to unstable work situations. Diversity provides protection against changing circumstances.

Though much of this chapter describes the ways an individual can cope with many difficult changes in work and life, our emphasis is ultimately positive. As we have seen, interesting and difficult work enables us to carry our mental vigor well into our senior years—far more than the people who have a single, comfortable job all their lives. Someone with a general set of cognitive and learning skills can successfully adapt to new work situations and also *enjoy* the challenge of such changes. The research I did in the medical library was the best three weeks of my life.

===== **LESSONS IN BRAINPOWER** =====

- We must work to develop enough kinds of knowledge to protect ourselves from the unpredictability of life. Developing the broad mental skills of a generalist gives us the best opportunity for surviving in a complex and ever-changing world.
- Multidisciplinary approaches work not only because new people bring fresh ideas to a situation but also because new perspectives draw the usual decision makers out of their old mind-sets so that they contribute new ideas, too.
- Being able to approach a problem from a variety of mental perspectives is like having a panel of experts in our head, each of whom asks different questions about the problem. It can lead us to insights that would not otherwise be possible.

FIFTEEN

Education for Change

If a vital, multifaceted career keeps our brain in good shape, we must be prepared for such a career. Early training will help our children be more open to and less threatened by change. They need to be ready because life often presents us with unexpected disruptions and circumstances that are beyond our control. These may be minor, such as routine but difficult work or family circumstances; or they may be major, such as personal catastrophes or major upheavals in the economy. The world is a mess, full of "noise" and chaos. Chance plays a role in everyone's life. It was chance that saved my mother's life under the Nazi regime and chance that took my father's. It was chance that led us out of Czechoslovakia in 1949, just before the fall of the Iron Curtain. It was chance that put me under the tutelage of a wonderful teacher who stimulated my lifelong love of learning. It was chance that made me part of the original class of sixteen students when the first psychology degree program was launched in Israel. It was chance that led me into politics. The deputy prime minister had been a student of mine and we became friends. When he became prime minister, we talked from time to time about the unique pressures of running our nation's government. One day he called me and said, "Would you consider changing your life for a while? There's an election in three months . . ."

To a large degree, it was also chance that led me to found CogniFit. After seeing the early PET brain scans in 1983, I continued to follow the field. Every time I read a new article about the way the brain adapts (can be trained) as the result of mental stimuli and challenges, I set the information aside in a folder. Even while pursuing my own separate studies, I remained fascinated by the unfolding revelations about the brain's ability to alter both function and form. The research fell into the category of interesting things that we happen not to pursue. Many years later, when the government created a program to incubate new science businesses in Israel, I was asked whether I had any ideas. Out came the folder. I realized that in the two decades that had passed since the first brain scans, the science had made it—matured enough to be unquestioned in its conclusions. And personal computers had evolved from hobbyist toys to sophisticated tools that were widely available. Plus, a social shift had occurred. The elderly no longer expected to sit on a bench and watch the world go by. Baby Boomers were beginning to transform the common perceptions of aging. They were far more active and engaged in the world than previous generations, and they wanted to stay fit in every way. All of the elements had emerged that were necessary for crafting a serious cognitive training program. The government chose to help seed this venture—a risky idea, because the company would be among the first of its kind anywhere in the world.

No doubt many other business and personal adventures begin by similar serendipity—the confluence of interest, preparation, and luck.

Being ready to cope with chance when it is negative or take advantage of it when it is positive requires cognitive flexibility. Children and young adults have a natural curiosity. The best way to take advantage of this trait and give them the tools they need to take on our ever-challenging world may be to return to a more classical approach to education. In the West, a classical education meant just that: study of the classic works of history, science, and literature, often in the original Greek or Latin. Plutarch's *Lives,* which paired biographies of famous Greeks and Romans with an emphasis on character, is an excellent book from many perspectives: literary, historical, political, legal, and ethical. It should be required reading for any college student or cultured person, as it once was, and not merely the purview of scholars of the classical epoch in Western history.

Since World War II, the movement in education has been mostly toward more and more specialization. Relatively few schools still teach the classics, or have other broad curricula designed to expand the mind. Our education systems tend to focus on the scientific way of thinking, with a little bit of literary and historical thought thrown in. That's about it. This is a grave mistake. A narrow education and occupational specialization put a person in jeopardy both professionally and cognitively. The benefit of a broader education is that, although we learn less about one particular subject, we learn more about many subjects. We develop different underlying learning skills and the ability to apply multiple ways of thinking to a variety of situations.

Plowing through the dense works of the ancients does not likely appeal to many people, and the turgid and punitive methods by which the classical education was often dispensed is equally unappealing. Yet the traditional education aimed to create generalists, enlightened adults capable of taking a broad view of the world. Beneficiaries of this education lived during a time of great advancements in science, literature, art, and exploration. The West was developing technology that was as cutting edge for those eras as our technology is to us. Adventurers canvassed the world with an energy that had not been seen since prehistoric times. Graduates of the classical universities were expected to have the versatility to take on any number of roles: writers, artists, scientists, explorers, clergy, government (and colonial) ministers, diplomats or warriors, and (indirectly) businessmen. The broad-based set of skills needed then is just as applicable today.

One criticism of the traditional approach is that it limits our study to the culture and biases of "dead white guys"—well-educated, aristocratic males of European ancestry. By eliminating the outdated material from the classical approach, we make room to teach students the best of the present along with the best of the past. We can offer enough of our traditional teaching to give students a strong taste of Western thought and ethics, without overwhelming them with the in-depth coursework in the classics that marked earlier generations of education.

This type of curriculum works regardless of whether students are fully a part of that European-centric culture or not. The Barclay Elementary and Middle School, a poor black public school in Baltimore, turned the educational world on its head in the 1990s when it ditched its modern curriculum de jour and partnered with a wealthy white private school to teach a classical curriculum that in most ways had not been updated in more than a hundred years. Student scores at Barclay rose from the 20th percentile, typical of inner-city schools, to the 50th percentile. Language scores doubled from below the 30th percentile to above the 60th. Another combination of diverse topics studied rigorously would likely have resulted in similar improvements, though immersion in the mainstream American cultural thought provided opportunities of particular value to these minority students.

Exposing students to a broad range of interests will raise their curiosity level in general. Students should be given enough of a grounding that they are stimulated to pursue some of the topics independently. If they are not exposed to them in school, the chances are very small that they will come to them later on in life. This is something of a cafeteria approach, giving students a taste of many different things to pique their interest while they're still young. Not a superficial scanning, mind you, but enough to engage the mind.

Part of the cafeteria approach *must be* exposure to cultures other than our own. We have plenty of opportunities to expand educational diversity in schools and with it bring new ways of thinking. Including the study of other heritages is not the same as eliminating the study of Western heritage. The same is true of education in Arabic, Asian, African, or other cultures. They need not toss out their own heritage in order to include others.

Many of today's small liberal arts colleges strive to provide the varied curriculum discussed here, and students who take advantage of different *kinds* of subjects emerge well prepared to deal with our modern world. But few schools push students outside of their majors or their comfort zones. Most students stay within related domains of thought—literature, history, and sociology, for instance, or math and chemistry and physics, but the objective is not to pile on more of the same. Every university degree should strive to pair work in different and seemingly incompatible fields. Schools might require, for instance, that every English major have a science minor, or vice versa. The more disparate subjects the student studies, the better.

EDUCATION FOR CHANGE

My colleague Betty Friedan once described this new way of teaching as "changeducation": a restructuring of education to help people deal with change, an approach that will help them develop and maintain their cognitive reserves well into adulthood. Parents and teachers tend to teach one way of doing things. Most children still experiment—and they are sometimes punished for it. We need to take advantage of the child's naturally playful brain. This requires us to dispense with curricula that are designed to help students pass proficiency examinations or meet certain standards of knowledge. The goal should be to get beyond single-answer, factual questions or "always true" answers. How much is one plus one? What are the major geographic features of our home state? Knowing the answers to such questions is necessary but it isn't enough to help us develop the mental skills we need for life.

Complex questions that lead to "sometimes true" answers, and conditional questions that may have multiple answers according to the circumstances, are far more mentally challenging. Exposure to these types of questions will help students build their brainpower and avoid cognitive automatic pilot. A new curriculum will be good for teachers as well. Teaching the same subjects the same way year after year, they tend to burn out. Providing creative new ways to teach will help teachers avoid routine and rigid approaches to teaching.

A valuable new class might focus on how to develop and maintain relationships. Learning more about their self-perception, how others perceive them, and how to treat others would help students gain emotional intelligence. It would not be a "feel good" approach in which everyone is supposed to like one another at the end. (Not that learning to play nice would be a bad outcome.) The goal would be to give students the skills to manage relationships, *especially* those that are difficult. Or how about a class that teaches strategies on avoiding automaticity? Perhaps we could construct a curriculum based on the many examples in this book, equipping students with the tools they need to maintain mental flexibility.

These types of changes will be difficult to implement in cultures focused on standard achievement tests in core subjects, which is currently the direction being taken in the United States and elsewhere. But it is not impossible. With a slight shift in emphasis from total scores to student improvement year by year, the educational system can eliminate many of the shortcomings of the current approach as well as lay the groundwork for students doing better in the long term across a broader range of subjects. Anyone doubting the need for a redesign of education might benefit from a recent study, *Academically Adrift: Limited Learning on College Campuses,* by sociologists Richard Arum and Josipa Roksa. The book found that 45 percent of today's college students show no significant improvement in critical thinking, complex reasoning, and writing skills after two years of college. More than one-third fail to improve after four years of college. *Students showing the greatest gains were the ones who had read and written the most and who had taken the traditional liberal arts education.*

SOMETIMES TRUE, ALWAYS TROUBLING

Ethical problems are good examples of multi-answer or "sometimes true" situations. In an ethical problem, each possible solution is a compromise, and each compromise raises as many questions as it does answers. Often the resolution means choosing between the lesser of two evils. Even then, rational people can disagree about which choice is preferable.

Some people refuse to consider more than one side to an ethical dilemma, dismissing the "sometimes true" as "situational ethics," in which we alter our principles to fit the circumstance. In reality, life regularly brings our various principles into conflict, as the following examples show. That some people resist fully engaging in ethical dilemmas is an indication of just how difficult such questions can be and how much cognitive effort is needed to tackle them.

It does not help that ethicists tend to pose ethical dilemmas that few of us will ever face. It is unlikely that many of us will have to choose whether to kill another passenger on a sinking ship so we can get the last life vest. It is even less likely that we will find five people tied to a track and the only way of saving them is to throw a sixth under the train to stop it. It is pretty certain that none of us will have the opportunity to go back in time where we can decide whether to kill an innocent child by the name of Adolf Hitler.

Though such questions may be useful for deep thinkers who wish to ponder philosophical matters, most of us face much more immediate and practical ethical choices in our everyday lives. A topic that arises regularly for advice columnists, for instance, is the question of what to do when we find out that someone is cheating on his or her romantic partner. Some people believe that the injured party should always be told. Others believe the opposite, that people should always mind their own business. People on opposite sides of the question are likely to get into heated debate. Do circumstances matter? What if we know the indiscretion was a one-time mistake—that the person repents and now treats his or her partner wonderfully? Is it less of an issue if the two principals are not formally engaged? Is it more of an issue if they plan to get married in a month? It often happens that the aggrieved party does not believe the accusation or blames the messenger. Do we factor into the equation the possible harm to our friendship? If we work with one or both parties, should our decision hinge on whether speaking up could cost us our job? Does it balance the scales if the aggrieved party has also cheated? Again, some people may come down firmly for A or B without any second-guessing. Most people, however, would weigh all of these factors before making their decision.

Genetic testing also raises many difficult ethical questions. On the social, political, and legal level is the question of how the genetic information might be used if it's made publicly available. (In the United States, employers and insurers cannot discriminate against anyone on the basis of genetic information—at least in theory.) On the personal level is the question of our right to know about our medical condition versus the possible impact of that knowledge. Huntington's is an example of a disease that can cause such a dilemma. Currently incurable, it is a degenerative disease of the brain cells caused by a defective gene. (A dominant gene, it needs to be inherited from only one parent.) Knowing that we will die in ten or twenty years can devastate the rest of our lives. We have a right *not* to know. If our parent has Huntington's, we face the choice of taking a test to determine whether we may have it, too. If we're young and test positive for Huntington's, still more ethical issues arise. The first is whether we should have children, since every child will have a 50 percent chance of inheriting the fatal disease. The second is what we tell our parents if they do not already know their status. One of them must also have it; being older, they will begin to suffer sooner. Should they be told so that they have time to get their affairs in order and prepare for the onset of the terrible disease? Should they be spared for as long as possible?

If we are the one who has the knowledge, the decision to tell or not to tell could depend on a subjective assessment of the personality and character of our relatives. Do we think they would be harmed more by knowing, or by not knowing? The decision might also involve the age, health, and lifestyle of the affected parties.

The United States has developed a program that handles issues relating to Huntington's, including opening a few testing centers. Professional support is provided for people who learn that they have the disease. The doctor who runs the program had a parent who died of Huntington's. She has never had herself tested. She would rather not know, but she has devoted her entire adult life to seeking a cure for the disease.

The more genetic tests we develop, the more often we will find ourselves facing these types of paradoxes. In addition to a medical directive that tells doctors what to do in matters relating to our physical health, we may also need a psychological medical directive that describes what kind of diseases we want to be told about and what kinds we do not.

Let's explore another ethical conflict. Currently, researchers are experimenting with drugs that may have the power to prevent the laying down of memories or to dissolve ones that already exist. A woman might receive this kind of drug to prevent the formation of the long-term memory of a rape or another type of assault. Soldiers suffering from post-traumatic stress might be able to shed their haunting memories. But do we then take a pill to erase every unhappy occurrence—the perfect "happy pill"? Many of the unpleasant memories of our past help make us who we are. Do we reserve such treatments for people who are suffering after specific kinds of violent trauma? If the memory involves an attack, what of the person accused of the crime, who has the right to be confronted by his or her accuser? How can the accuser testify if the memory of the event has been wiped? Freeing the victim from suffering might endanger society's ability to put away the perpetrator.

Perhaps the most difficult and troubling moral conflict that the average person might face is that of abortion. For this example, let's focus on the one scenario that creates an unquestionable moral conflict: the pregnant woman who contracts a potentially fatal disease. Many forms of cancer arise during pregnancy, including breast, melanoma, Hodgkins, ovarian, leukemia, colorectal, and choriocarcinoma—the last being caused by the pregnancy itself. Cancer is rare among pregnant women, affecting less than 1 percent. In many cases the disease can be managed in such a way that both the woman and the fetus can be saved. But with 6.7 million pregnancies a year in the United States alone, several thousand women a year face a terrible choice. Treating her cancer will kill the fetus. Not treating the cancer will kill her. Still more women face this crippling decision because of other conditions, accidents, or trauma in which medical treatment for themselves will lead to the death of their fetuses.

Do we assume automatically that the mother should live? Do we automatically assume that the life of the fetus should take precedence? Many women might well choose to sacrifice themselves to save their unborn child. But ask the husband: Many men would chose to save their wife. Yet what if the mother wants to save herself and the father wants to save the child? What if the woman has other young children to whom the loss of a mother would be devastating?

In all the scenarios we've discussed, some few people would automatically choose A. Some would automatically choose B. Most thinking people, however, would weigh a number of factors—and still be torn over their final, agonizing decision. Approaching the question from several of the different mental perspectives might help. The scientific mode would weigh the kind of disease involved, where it is within the body, how advanced and aggressive it is, and how advanced the pregnancy is. (The earlier the treatment, the more danger there is to the fetus.) All of these factors bear on the relative risk to the mother and child posed by immediate versus delayed treatment. The legal mode would weigh the question of the legality of any action and whether legal precedent favored one over the other. The historical mode might try to understand how these diffi-cult decisions have been made throughout history and particularly in societies similar to our own. The ethical philosopher mode would try to weigh right versus wrong according to the ethical traditions of that person.

TEACHING BASED ON ETHICAL PROBLEMS

Difficult ethical questions are seldom addressed in the average schoolroom and are almost never presented before a student reaches college. Far too many young people finish high school without ever confronting an important issue with which they disagree. Often a teenager's views are the unthinking recapitulation of the views of their peers or parents rather than their own independent beliefs. They never have an opportunity to dive into the reasons for their support of one position or to examine the reasons for their objec-tions to another. They never get to dig into facts that might support or oppose their point of view. They never face tough questions that have more than one possible answer. The goal is not to encourage them to reject their existing points of view but to ensure that they have thought them through. Careful consideration may lead them to the same conclusions as their parents, for example, but it will give them a deeper understanding as to *why*. They will own their ideas, which is better than having inherited them. And they just may come away with more respect for the countervailing point of view. In Israel, many schools are reinstituting oratory classes and debat-ing clubs to give students the experience of being required to argue

a case by fully developing it according to formal and logical principles . . . and then to argue the same case from opposing points of
view.

Another element of the ethical dilemma is the question of whether
to focus on intention or the end result. Jean Piaget, the Swiss psychologist who pioneered the study of cognitive development in children, regularly posed the following scenario to his young charges.
One boy, in trying to help his mother, drops and breaks ten glasses.
Another boy, told not to touch a glass, does so anyway and breaks
it. Which boy deserves more punishment? Until the age of about ten
or eleven, most children would say that the boy who breaks the
most glasses should be punished more. They cannot distinguish between intent and result. (A contributing factor for young children is
that they perceive that a parent would be angrier if ten glasses were
broken rather than one.)

As children approach the age of twelve, they begin to recognize
that intent matters, and their answers shift to the other side. Piaget's
studies show that at this age children begin to develop the ability to
perform "formal operations." They can learn rules of logic such as
those involving mathematics and science, and they can abstract behavioral principles from the situations they encounter. One of the
core principles is that of intent, which is an important element in
society and in law. The difference between murder and manslaugh-
ter is whether the perpetrator intended to harm the victim. In certain crimes, intent has to be proven before a crime is even considered
to have been committed. Yet the law considers the end results, too.
A person who kills someone in a car wreck will generally get a
harsher penalty than if the wreck caused only an injury.

Ethical dilemmas take us far beyond our comfort zones. Our
first step to adulthood is to recognize that we can form principles
and that these principles can guide us through many situations. The
second step is to recognize that there are exceptions to how we
apply principles. The complexity of life punches holes in our ability
to uniformly apply principles and laws. It is not that we change our
principles out of convenience. Because life does not deliver problems in neat and tidy boxes, we are confounded when we try to keep
all of our answers in neat and tidy boxes. We might apply the same

principle in two different situations and come out with different decisions. Or, we apply principle A rigorously only to discover that our action causes us to violate principle B, which we hold just as dear. Or vice versa.

Our brains appear to have "exception circuits" built in. In trying to determine the most efficient computational strategy the brain might employ, MIT's Marvin Minsky posited that the simplest way to handle a "sometimes true" rule is not to dismantle the original rule or create multiple rules. Rather, the solution is to wire the primary rule to designated exceptions. We can apply the rule confidently when normal conditions apply but flag unusual circumstance that might change the result. The consideration of all possible options and points of view when confronted with an ethical dilemma must have the effect of strengthening the brain circuits when the rule does apply, while also increasing the branches that are made to handle the few exceptions when it does not. The net result is an increase in cognitive power and agility.

Very few things in life are as clear-cut as math. Ethical dilemmas are one example of the complexity in the world. These types of questions require the brain to first abstract a principle and then develop the ability to see when, how, and to what extent we can apply it while balancing contradictory principles. Being a good friend to one person could mean totally different behavior than being a good friend to another. Not because we change the principle of being a good friend but because different people need different things from us. One friend might need to be encouraged to be more adventurous; another might need to be cautioned against excessive risk-taking. One friend might need someone to talk to and want to hear our thoughts; another might bristle at our advice. Parenting would be the easiest job in the world if all children thought the same way, behaved the same way, behaved consistently (!), and responded to discipline in the same way. In confronting the complexity of these and other problems, the mind has to remain open, to experiment, to understand how many important matters depend on the nuances of circumstance, relationship, and individuality.

To train the brain from childhood about the importance of details and context is the opposite of satisfycing. Rather than seeking a similarity that leads to a quick answer, we seek a difference that causes us to think afresh. This new way of learning will also bestow us with the ability to delay judgment, to postpone an immediate reaction to new information so that we can be sure to gather all the facts and avoid automatic, simplistic ways of looking at things. Only in this way can we apply mature, considered judgment to the bewildering problems in life. Here is the beginning of wisdom.

═══ LESSONS IN BRAINPOWER ═══

- Modern life is so full of chaos and chance that we must all be prepared for almost anything. This requires cognitive flexibility.
- Achieving cognitive flexibility requires an education designed to investigate problems at a deep level and to teach several different modes of thought. It is not enough to take difficult classes; we need classes that exercise the brain in dramatically different ways.
- Learning to tackle complex issues such as ethical dilemmas will improve thinking skills *and results* on achievement tests while laying a much deeper cognitive foundation for life. Complex questions that have "sometimes true" answers are the most cognitively stimulating, because they require us to delve into detail, nuance, and context.

— PART V —

THINKING AHEAD

SIXTEEN

Too Ancient for Our Lives

Several years ago . . .

As I drive, something to the side of the road catches my atten-tion. Peripheral vision cannot see clearly but it compels the brain to attend. Wired to be vigilant for predators or prey, we are naturally alert to any movement around us. Quickly weighing the risk of looking to the side versus the risk of looking away from the front, the brain decides to move the eyes or the head, possibly both. In the next few dozen milliseconds, my eyes per-ceive a pattern of light, shade, and color. More milliseconds pass as my brain interprets the patterns to be a boy and a ball, both partly obscured by a vehicle.

Comparing the boy and the ball to the stationary car, my brain continues to perceive relative movement. Realizing that the ball is bouncing toward the street with the boy in hot pur-suit, I make complex ballistic calculations. At my current speed, will I pass in front of or behind him or will we collide? Given my relative position, do I try to stop, hit the accelerator to pass ahead, or swerve into the next lane? Have I checked recently enough to know whether the next lane is clear? Is there time to

honk so that the boy will stop? More dozens of milliseconds
pass as the brain processes these semiconscious thoughts.

The ball bounces into the street. I slam on the brakes. Tires
squeal. The boy races into the street. The car fishtails slightly but
stops. The boy grabs the ball and looks up. He is as astonished
at my apparition as I am at his. Reminded of the danger by the
sight of my bumper—a mere foot from where he stands—he
looks both ways and then continues across the road.

A second or two later, I realize that I have not run down a
careless seven-year-old. Heart pounding, hands shaking, I have
to pull over for a moment to recover my composure. That was
close, I think, having very nearly experienced the accident that
driving instructors warn about: a child's wild dash into the
street. I am torn between leaving quietly and finding the boy's
parents to tell them what has happened. Eventually I drive away,
figuring the child will remember the lesson on his own for quite
some time.

Anyone who has ever driven a car has likely experienced this
kind of horrifying near-miss: A car turns unexpectedly into our
path, a dangerous object falls off a truck, we hit a patch of invisible
ice and the car starts to slide sickeningly toward a vehicle coming
the other way. When the moment has passed and we realize that we
have survived, we all deal with the same heart-pounding aftermath
of relief and disbelief.

What we may not realize is that this physical reaction is not supposed to occur *after* the high-speed encounter. It's supposed to happen *before*. The surge of adrenaline, the racing heart and lungs, the
muscle tension: These "fight or flight" reactions evolved for action
that is already behind us! In most modern emergencies, the danger
has already passed or hit us by the time these responses kick in. The
boy faced the same predicament: He had already stepped into my
car's path by the time he heard the squealing tires. Animals likewise
have no defensive adaptation for a predator as fast as modern vehicles. Deer freeze when startled because in natural environments
their coloration render them nearly invisible when they're motion-
less. On the road—especially in front of headlights—they are ren-

dered helpless. Despite the brain's ability to perceive and react in terms of tenths of a second, despite the body's marvelous shortcuts to improve reaction time (think of the automatic reflex that causes us to yank our hand off a hot stove), our inventions have outrun the response times and adaptations of all living creatures, ourselves included. Humans are physiologically and cognitively obsolete for the world we have created.

Though we are probably the youngest species of any complexity on earth, we stand on the shoulders of all of the organisms that came before us. Our DNA stretches back to the time when the double strands first embraced. We are old stuff. Cognitively, we are too ancient for our lives in at least four ways:

1. Speed of information processing.
2. Nature of response.
3. Knowledge of the future.
4. Preoccupation with technology.

Speed of information processing. No one can accurately determine the average speed of mental processes. A single neuron can respond in a few thousandths of a second, but most reactions involve multiple neurons or clusters of neurons. Signals are transmitted by an electrochemical process that is fast compared to most natural actions but slow compared to an electronic transmission. For complex behaviors, our speed is more akin to parcel post than a telephone call.

We evolved in a world in which the fastest moving object was a creature on the run. Our reflexes cannot respond to anything that's faster than a moving bicycle. An automobile routinely goes three times as fast. Two vehicles approaching each other at highway speeds require reaction times ten times faster than what we're capable of. Our biology poses very real constraints, especially for new drivers. Younger drivers have quicker reflexes than their elders, but they have less driving experience. The basics are not yet automatic for them, so they have to attend to everything they do. This is why distractions, which are bad for any drivers, are particularly dangerous for them. It takes experience for the brain to learn how to properly estimate distance and speed. Evidence shows that it takes two years for this perceptual learning to take hold and for new drivers to improve and become safer.

Because our command-and-control centers are not fully mature until our twenties, teenagers are more prone to risky behavior. Traffic accidents are their leading cause of death. Fatalities are often fueled by alcohol or a failure to use seat belts. And of course by cellphones, which raise accident rates as much as alcohol use does. Most states now have graduated licenses for young drivers that, among other restrictions, do not permit cellphone use or late-night driving and limit the number of other teenagers allowed in the car. The most comprehensive graduated licensing programs have reduced fatal crashes among sixteen-year-olds by 20 percent.

The relative inaccuracy and slow speed of human thought has other effects. Financial trading systems are now so fast and complex that few people (if any) can manage them or even explain exactly how they work. If a trader errs or responds too slowly in Singapore, the stock markets in New York may experience wild swings. Even in retrospect, it's hard to grasp the role that automated systems played in the recent financial meltdowns. When one software trading program sets off another software trading program, humans pretty much have to wait until the cascading effect is over to assess the monetary carnage.

A similar problem is now prompting a battlefield debate. Computerized weapon systems that are currently under development range from ever more sophisticated flying drones to rolling machine-gun platforms. The military wants these robotic systems to reduce the danger to soldiers, improve speed, and provide a rational response under fire. Supporters of computerized weapons believe that machines will be better able to adhere to battlefield rules of engagement than soldiers, whose panic might lead to overreaction or civilian casualties. Opponents fear that the use of machines in place of people will reduce the human cost of combat, thereby lowering the threshold for starting wars. No doubt there is also at least a subliminal fear of the oft-writ science-fiction scenario of thinking machines that take over the world.

Nature of response. Not only are we too slow to react to many modern challenges, but we are also wired to react in the *wrong* way. Having evolved in a physical world, our responses are of a physical nature. Adrenaline surges enable us to run faster, jump higher, or hit harder. We've all heard stories about heroes who have lifted victims out from under extraordinary weights or saved people from raging fires, but most of the time human responses are inappropriate to modern emergencies. The nature of most threats has changed from physical to mental. When meeting an important client or interviewing for a job, the last thing we want is to engage our "fight or flight" response, yet here we are with a racing pulse and sweating palms. A fear response inhibits our ability to think, recall important information, and improvise. If our boss yells at us, we are not likely to earn a promotion by pummeling him. Police officers, who are asked to face frightening situations daily without responding by instinct, rely on their training and experience to keep their professional cool. When an officer breaks down and strikes out in response to a provocation, we hear cries of "police brutality!" rather than "biological contradiction!" Automatic reflexes can be counterproductive in an emergency that requires a measured response.

The stress response itself, which was covered in detail earlier, is yet another example of a mismatch between biology and modern life. We are wired to respond to a relatively few but highly dangerous situations in the physical world. We are *not* wired to respond day after day, year after year, to psychological stress—which the body interprets as a physical threat. Hypertension is the likely result of mild but prolonged stress. The effectiveness of our vascular system depends on the ability of blood vessels to contract and expand as physical stress rises and falls. Prolonged stress reduces the flexibility of the vessels. The only way for the heart to deliver the volume of blood that's needed is to pump harder, raising blood pressure to potentially dangerous levels. Our circulatory system is designed for one kind of life. We are living another.

Another way in which we are maladapted is our sensitivity to social slights. Historically, we lived in small, tightly integrated groups that were leery of outsiders. Our life and livelihood depended on cooperation within our tribe or clan. Social interactions were intense. Our ability to get along with others could make the difference between getting food and getting exiled. Now we have far more social interactions with far more people, and most of these interactions are superficial. I am often asked about the difficulty most of us have with remembering names. I say, "You know too many people!" Historically, we needed to remember only forty to fifty names. Now we are expected to remember hundreds or even thousands—including the names of people we might have met just once.

Shallow or not, routine social interactions can affect our minds as much as if our very survival were at stake. As a result, we are unbelievably vulnerable to the slightest bit of nonsense from other people. A rude remark from a passerby or a catty comment made by a coworker, and our day is ruined. The explosive potential of this social sensitivity can be seen in road rage and fights over parking spaces. Psychologically, we respond to the first as if we are being assaulted and the second as if someone is trying to snatch the game we killed.

Knowledge of the future. Humans have pondered our mortality for as long as we have existed. The contents of prehistoric graves indicate that we have also always believed in, or at least hoped for, a world beyond this one. The brain has the ability to project its demise and conceive of more pleasant alternatives. It is likely that we (and possibly our Neanderthal cousins) are the only species to consider the future and what it might bring. And we are almost certainly the only species to plan and build for an existence beyond our own life spans. We need look no further than the opulent tombs of the ancient Egyptians, well-stocked with provisions and treasures; the lofty cathedrals built by Christians; and, to consider more modern examples, the business empires and trust funds that moguls leave to their heirs.

Whereas other species might be able to perceive enough of the future to predict the location of food or the changing of the seasons, we can forecast storms, weather patterns, and even climate change. We can predict the outbreak of diseases and the outcome of elections. The most alert among us can predict financial collapses (which the rest of us ignore until it is too late!). And our ability to estimate our life span and the most likely cause of our future demise will only increase as we learn more about genetics. This growing ability to foresee our fate well in advance is both sobering and unsettling. Increasingly refined knowledge of our mortality provides more grist for our internal worry mills, raising the stress on our hypertensive hearts and accentuating our maladaptation to life.

Preoccupation with technology. The impact of the flood of digital downloads among today's "hip" generation might best be described by a movie title: *The Invasion of the Mind Snatchers.* Not only are tech lovers switching data feeds constantly, disrupting the brain's ability to form lasting memories, but these users are also relying on digital devices for longer and longer stretches of time. What used to be a few moments of serenity at the bus stop are now consumed with mobile games. Our need for external stimulus is balanced by a need for quiet. The brain needs time for reflection so that it can assimilate and organize all of the information that's pouring in. Whether in the form of contemplation or actual dreams, the brain needs downtime to contemplate, to decide what information is worth keeping, and how it relates to our past experiences and memories.

The brain also needs genuine information, not just sound bites and visual feeds. *The Last Child in the Woods* is a book that examines the very real fear that many of today's children will never stroll among pine trees, experience wildlife, or inhale the scents of the natural world. Human experience continues its slide toward urban life and technology. The cognitive damage, not to mention the cultural loss, caused by isolation from nature is incalculable. People learn better after a walk in nature than after a walk in a busy city, because there are fewer distractions. Streaming feeds of nature "live" to a computer screen or TV monitor will never compare with the whole-body sensory input that comes from a walk in the woods. Photos, videos, and alphanumeric symbols are thin gruel compared to the real world encountered directly.

It's even more important for us to experience frequent face-to-face communication with other humans. One of the key ways in which we learn to interact is by mimicking physical movements and expressions and by relating body language to the meaning of the words being spoken. We do not simply respond to information but to the context in which it is presented. Imagine the peril of a world in which humans are unable to read intent through facial expressions and body language, and all of the other emotional subtexts of personal engagement, because we have so little practice in physical contact. One teenager gave up texting as an experiment. In reconnecting directly with her peers, she realized that her smartphone had nearly eliminated face time with her girlfriends. Today's adults can correctly assess one another's emotion almost all of the time. Research shows that teenagers are correct only half the time. If they are seldom face-to-face, how will young people improve their ability to gauge one another's psychological state?

Another issue is that the torrent of digital information will addict the brain. Just as a thoughtful person yearns for a reprieve from information overload and feels pain when it does not relent, a digital wonk yearns for more data when the onslaught stops and feels pain when the information spigot clamps shut. Unquestionably, the brain will adapt. But the adaptation will be in the form of shutting down deeper and more complex thought, failing to store as much data or to make complex connections, falling back on instant and primitive defense mechanisms. Imagine the peril of a world in which a growing number of humans revert to stereotypical responses to new information, people, and cultures because they have lost the ability to process any significant amount of sophisticated information. History is replete with irony. The biggest irony could be that technical developments first enabled the expansion of our inner world and later drowned it out. Will the legacy of the digital era be the elevation of ignorance?

IN SEARCH OF BALANCE

Sounding an alarm about the dangers of digital technology is not the same thing as rejecting that technology. Every technology can be, and has been, used for good and ill. Modern modes of transportation can speed the delivery of goods and services or of bombs and missiles. Modern physics can provide clean energy or a dirty end to civilization. Even technology intended for good can create harm. Most modern conveniences are powered by environmentally harmful fossil fuels that could disrupt the very lifestyle they brought into being. Modern medicine can eliminate most diseases and also create virulent new ones.

It is not a bad thing that machines have reduced life's physical challenges. We would all rather exercise in our leisure time than suffer through twelve hours of backbreaking labor. Nor is it a bad thing that new kinds of machines are reducing life's mental challenges. New technology can easily handle the complexity that used to be foisted upon humans. No one really wants to do long ledgers of calculations by hand in order to keep our brains sharp. Except for hobbyists, no one wants to bring back early computers because they require more mental effort by the user. We want to take advantage of all the power that our modern systems have to tackle difficult challenges, including the solving of certain problems that would take decades to do by hand. This book was created largely through online research and collaboration, reducing the time of completion by a year or more compared to traditional methods. If we use digital devices to handle our problems more easily, we must simply recognize that this convenience comes at a cognitive price that must be offset by a cognitive effort elsewhere, whether through a brain-training regimen or through other difficult mental tasks. (Training can complement and build upon the other effortful work we do elsewhere in our lives. It cannot replace life activities that engage our minds on a deep level, such as immersion in a project or a good book. What it can do is ensure that our brains do not get lazy.)

Those of us who oppose texting while driving are not opposed to smartphones. We are opposed to drivers (mostly young ones) being killed in automobile accidents. Those of us who raise concerns about multitasking are not opposed to the proliferation of data. We are opposed to misconceptions that lead to a reduction rather than an increase in learning. Those of us who call for a respite from digital noise are not opposed to digital devices any more than those who oppose ear-splitting decibel levels are opposed to music. They are opposed to hearing loss; we are opposed to brain loss.

For people who work at home or travel constantly, digital tools such as Skype and email reduce the sense of isolation. Technology allows people who are physically distant to share ideas, brainstorm, and collaborate. The digital world can create new and exciting realities and take us to places that it would otherwise be impossible for us to go. Only twelve men have ever walked on the face of the moon. No one has ventured to Mars or beyond. Yet technology has enabled millions of people to become virtual explorers of far-off moons and planets. Digital technology has the unique ability to show us universes that are astronomically too large, infinitesimally too small, or environmentally too extreme for humans to explore. It can also give us access to places that are just too expensive for the average person to go. In these situations, the choice is not between a full and faux experience but between a faux experience and no experience at all. If the object of the digital lifestyle is to saturate the brain, our object must be to ensure that this does not happen—that we are disciplined enough to accept only what is valuable.

Society has never rejected anything it perceives as progress, but it is possible that the "all digital, all the time" mind-set could lead to a backlash. Just as some people reject urban life for the quiet countryside and some towns ban vehicles to provide a more enjoyable environment for pedestrians, some communities may insist upon having islands of sanity that ban cellphones and other intrusive devices. All of Africa has cellphone reception, yet there are places in the Berkshires that lack coverage. The locals seem to be in no hurry to correct the oversight. People enjoying a quiet meal in a restaurant already find digital pollution as offensive as smoke pollution. Perhaps the digerati will be required to step outside with the smokers if they want to talk on their phones. No doubt certain communities will enjoy the status of being places where people can reflect on life rather than talk about it. Throw in a mud bath and massage, and we'll have a new kind of resort. (In fact, silent yoga retreats, with silent meditation ranging from a few days to many months, are gaining in popularity.)

Already, the brain has demonstrated the ability to receive and interpret electrical signals from physical prosthetics of various kinds. Philosophers are beginning to talk of cognitive prosthetics that will be no different than artificial limbs or cochlear implants. The phrase "cognitive prosthetic" might cover everything from software that helps train people with mild brain impairment to methods for organizing many different kinds of digital information to an extension of the mind that incorporates the processing power of external digital devices. In any of these scenarios, the singular principle is this: Anything that provides the brain with new, challenging information will expand our cognitive capabilities. Anything that offsets what we do with our brains, or provides only quick, short, superficial involvement, will reduce our cognitive capabilities. Anything that operates nonstop will fry our cognitive capabilities.

The potential to connect the brain to new mechanisms is another example of the way in which humans are becoming increasingly obsolete. Despite the brain's brilliance, we are not fast enough for modern life. The most intellectually advanced species on the planet is backward in comparison to the demands of its own life. At the same time that we are being cognitively spoiled by gadgets and by our relatively soft existence, the world in which we live presents ever-increasing demands on our mental abilities. We need to invest in cognition because the world is running away from us as a species. We need to work harder in order to prevent the ease of digital access to information from causing us to backslide mentally. We need to stay cognitively fit in order to better understand and prepare for an ever more rapid inculcation of technology into our lives. We must be wise enough to ensure that inventions do not constrain the brain but instead provide new ways to harness and enhance its abilities.

═══ LESSONS IN BRAINPOWER ═══

- Because our culture and our technology have advanced faster than we can advance biologically, human beings have become cognitively obsolete in the world we ourselves created!
- Our biology prepares us for an active physical reaction to the world, but most of the situations in modern life require a composed mental response.
- Our ability to predict the future—up to and including our own demise—renders us vulnerable to worry and stress.
- Our preoccupation with technology tends to isolate us from the natural world while addicting us to the ever-faster tempo and instant gratification provided by digital devices.
- The cognitive ease of the digital lifestyle means we need to consciously stimulate our minds.

SEVENTEEN

Sailors Passing Through a Port

The lifestyles of a farmer living in a small village and of a business-man living in the city differ in more respects than just their voca-tions and addresses. Both may have families with significant personal ties, but that's where the social similarity ends. The farmer is sur-rounded by a small, permanent group of people with whom he typ-ically interacts on a daily basis. He knows them by name and is intimately familiar with their personal histories. By contrast, the urbanite may see hundreds of people every day whom he will prob-ably never meet again. He learns to keep his distance, taking small, gradual steps to get to know neighbors and coworkers. After he fi-nally makes a few friends, he could well be transferred to another town, where he has to start again from scratch.

In a competitive, fast-moving society, it is difficult to turn down opportunities for advancement. Besides, how do we measure the advantages of a promotion, more significant and likely more inter-esting work, a higher standard of living, and the chance to meet new people against the cost of losing our existing colleagues, friends, and neighbors? Big opportunities usually involve a major disconti-nuity. It almost always seems preferable to take the plunge than to opt for slow advancement in a permanent position.

Some professions, or large companies within a profession, require extensive travel, regular relocation, or both. Jobs such as business consulting and military service require many months away from home at a time. The movie *Up in the Air* celebrates both the freedom and emptiness of a life transacted in airplanes, hotels, and conference rooms. In addition to raising stress levels, extended time away from home or actual relocation makes it difficult for people to develop social ties or nourish close family relationships.

The demands on our time are reaching new highs. Striking a good balance between work, family, leisure, and friends has never been easy. The problem becomes almost impossible as our jobs become ever more demanding. While domestic duties have become more of a shared burden in the Western world, women still bear the brunt, and are constantly in the position of juggling work and home. Only professional women with the resources to hire nannies have been able to approximate the career success of their male counterparts, yet many of them struggle with guilt over leaving so much child rearing to the hired help. The restraints on single men and women, with limited social ties, are obviously much smaller.

NO REST FOR THE WEARY

A traditional subsistence life, whether in the Middle Ages or today, is difficult and dangerous, but it does not necessarily require long hours—less than five hours a day of hard labor. The Industrial Revolution brought with it long work hours, six days a week, in unhealthy and unsafe sweatshops. Workers considered it a major victory when *child* labor was capped at twelve hours. Labor reform, especially after World War II, cut the workweek in half in most developed countries, to at or below forty hours a week.

Since then, this number has been steadily rising. During its ascension as a major economic power, Japan led the industrial nations in hours worked. Now, the United States has reclaimed that dubious distinction, averaging around 1,900 hours per person annually, or more than seven hours per workday. Nearly a full workweek was added during the decade of the 1990s alone. Only countries transitioning from "developing" to "developed" such as South Korea and

India work longer days. Americans, by the way, are the most productive workers in the world *per person,* but Europeans are the most productive on an hourly basis.

A whole field of study on work-life balance has sprung up, both on how to help individuals succeed professionally without abandoning their family and social lives and how to help companies retain highly productive employees who are not willing to sacrifice everything for their jobs. Nonetheless, those with the weakest personal commitments—usually the young and single (or at least childless)—have a clear competitive advantage. Those who choose a social and family life are seldom able to aggressively pursue the best career opportunities or are unwilling to upend their families for a few thousand bucks of increased pay. Employees on the fast track for promotion are the ones willing to literally get up and go.

This advantage ultimately alters the dynamics for senior business leaders. Historically, the people in these positions had a deep commitment to their companies and played major roles in their communities. Having risen through the ranks in society as well as in their companies, they were deeply invested in their corporate and social environments. Today, we run the risk that the new leadership represents people without significant ties to family, friends, or to the very organizations they serve. One school of executive coaching believes that CEOs should take the same kind of personality tests required of people in law enforcement in order to weed out the charming sociopaths who can easily rise through the ranks of business today.

More than one company has experienced the CEO who has come in, rung up huge profits, and left on his golden parachute, only for shareholders to later find out that the short-term profitability came at the expense of longer-term investments in vital areas such as research and development. The infamous behavior of CEOs who brought down entire companies such as Enron and WorldCom has been well-documented. "Liar loans" and a succession of other financial scams brought down an entire industry in 2008—and very nearly, the world's economic system. Is it a coincidence, or a remarkably long streak of bad luck, that so many of these large-scale frauds by dozens of once reputable companies are occurring now?

Or is it just the first fallout of having business leaders who lack roots?

Lack of commitment, of course, works both ways. Businesses now expect results faster than ever. If quarterly results are unsatisfactory, senior management is quickly out the door. This "what have you done for me lately" attitude is most apparent in sports, where coaches—even those who have won championships—are often fired after one or two poor seasons. Similarly, few CEOs are given the chance to establish success over the long term, even though the most thriving companies have CEOs who have been at the helm for years. As seen by steadily declining tenures in the "C suite," businesses and senior executives both seem to assume that any working relationship will be short. CEOs seek ever-larger compensation and severance packages, which protects them regardless of their performance, and corporations lavish cash and stocks on the next CEO in the hope of finding the white knight who will take the company to the top.

As a society, we seemed to be committed to a lack of commitment.

OPPORTUNISM VERSUS SOCIAL BONDS

Here now is the psychological problem: As social creatures, we have a highly developed need for bonding. This urge to form relationships, a drive we share with all other primates, is an integral part of our humanity. It is also an integral part of the development of our minds and identities. Our capacity for social bonding has enormous survival value and enhances our overall safety. From infancy we learn how to smile and ingratiate ourselves to others. Most childhood games involve learning social interaction as much as they do the development of some skill (for example, youth baseball). Traditional day-to-day life—hunting, working in fields, or sharing tasks inside the village—involves plenty of activities that bring people closer together. Except during the direst famine, traditional life also provides plenty of time for social activities and play. Under normal conditions, the bonds within the circle of extended family and friends continuously and almost automatically deepen. This ability to form close relationships is an extremely useful and well-honed skill that serves us throughout our entire life. However, the upward mobility of people who have shallow or no personal commitments can unravel social bonds.

Our predisposition for forming ever-deepening relationships has become a problem. The unraveling can be seen in three ways: 1) We cease to establish strong bonds. 2) We tend to treat relationships as being disposable. 3) We must struggle to develop relationships later on in life.

Pain is a powerful motivator for learning. To avoid the pain of severing personal relationships, we develop behaviors that prevent deep personal and social ties. Instead of forming long-term relationships, we "hook up" with no emotional attachment or have "friends with benefits." Online dating services are a sad commentary on the decline in social connections. The benefit of quickly finding someone with similar interests through online dating—or the somewhat more direct "speed dating"—is predicated on a lack of time to meet other people in normal and *safe* social settings. If freedom from commitment leads to professional advancement, more and more people are likely to avoid or delay it for as long as possible. Over the longer term this could cause the disruption of marriages and child-rearing.

Compounding our instinctive desire to avoid emotional pain is our desire to fit in—what is called normative pressure. Though we are inherently conservative, humans are also a social species—herd animals. Our conservatism means we feel safer with the pack than alone, so we can be stampeded into change when the pack moves on. In the modern world, our "safety in numbers" mind-set makes us susceptible to prevailing social trends, all sorts of fads, and consumerism. Advertisers, of course, are more than happy to play upon our psychological need to "keep up with the Joneses" in wealth, popularity, or couture. In modern society, normative pressure can make change the status quo! Change of fashion, as a way to remain a tribal member in good standing. Change of diet, as a solution to the failure of the current one. Change of spouse, as a way to overcome our marital problems. Change of car, of house, of location, and of lifestyle, as ways to achieve the ultimate goal of self-actualization. "You need change" is a frequent admonition from a friend. "I need change" is a frequent complaint when we describe our current malaise. Life is short, and change promises a quick fix to our difficulties.

The underlying cognitive principle is our increasingly low tolerance for routine. Constant change teaches the mind to seek yet more change. We are quickly bored. Repetition, any repetition, becomes intolerable in a relatively short amount of time. We have to feed our insatiable craving for stimulation. This permanent quest for novelty is cultivated by the media's strong emphasis on new things. To keep our attention from wandering, everything has to be highly interesting. The familiar and stable are stale.

Furthermore, in this age of consumerism, only mechanics from poor countries still repair things. If products fail, we throw them away and replace them with new ones. This mentality of disposability has spilled over into the personal domain as well. Rather than building a relationship and then doing the work of repairing it, we toss it aside the first time it sputters and begin looking for something new. We are becoming consumers of experience.

These points do not contradict the basic position that change is necessary to prevent mental stagnation and good in helping develop cognitive health. The danger comes when this thesis is carried too far. Recall the link between change and stress. Too much change brings as many problems as too little. Society as a whole can become fragmented by too many people seeking change too rapidly or in too many diverse ways. These pros and cons can be seen in globalization itself. It has devastated the workforces in many developed nations, particularly in the United States, but has also raised worldwide prosperity. In the 1960s, one-third of the world's nations supported the other two-thirds. Today, the reverse is true: two-thirds support the other one-third. Globalization and modern communications have also helped reduce the number of dictatorial regimes and continue to put pressure on the rest. Yet try to make these positive points to hard-working people who have lost their jobs to cheaper competitors overseas.

Stability remains the centerpiece of social norms. Conditions have to be sufficiently similar across time for us to develop coherent expectations about the way we should behave. Our minds need a reasonably consistent framework in order for us to make sense of reality. And some degree of permanence is needed to create a social consensus. If everything is in flux, if everyone is flying from one experience to the next, then the socializing effect of other people's behavior has a diminishing influence. In its extreme form, a lack of social norms can lead to chaos.

An absence of commitment to anything but career goals must, by necessity, include an absence of commitment to causes and ideals. But such hollow men and women, without principles and values, are the opposite of what we look for in positions of leadership. The strength of character of our leaders is more important to voters in democracies than any other virtues or skills that they may possess. The specter of the uncommitted poses a significant threat to the cohesion of modern society. The uncommitted are like sailors passing through a port. They are committed only to themselves. On a personal level, people who have learned to minimize their intimacy with others in order to advance their careers may realize one day that there is more to life fulfillment than a successful career. The problem is whether they can develop good relationships after so many years of avoiding them.

Not everyone who seeks change is an opportunist, of course. The United States in particular was settled by change seekers. The earliest settlers must have been highly motivated to migrate thousands of miles across the frigid lands and waters of the Arctic. Recent immigrants have chosen the New World over tyranny, injustice, religious persecution, poverty, or impossible family circumstances. Others simply set out to find their fortunes. Millions of people showed the courage to embrace change, and U.S. culture continues to encourage all things fresh and new. It is also possible, though by no means certain, that if tens of millions of people with similar exploratory traits all migrated to the same country and then intermarried over hundreds of years, that that country might have an inherited tendency toward change. Countries with large immigrant populations, such as the United States and Israel, have the most start-up companies. In Israel's case, it is not just in percentage terms but in absolute numbers. The small country has more start-up businesses than Britain, Germany, and France combined. Immigrant nations tend to be self-selected self-starters.

In general, change is encouraged and welcomed by some cultures and resisted by others. These change-a-phobic cultures often adopt the attitude: "If it's such a great idea, why hasn't anyone else already thought of it? If it doesn't exist, there must be a good reason." It's possible to generate an endless array of arguments about why it is not a good idea to start something new. In the world of medicine, researchers prefer scientists from certain countries when detailed and highly systematic testing needs to be done, while preferring scientists from other countries when more innovative approaches are required. A French magazine in the mid-1990s lamented that Bill Gates would never have been able to start Microsoft in France. The article listed a number of practical and cultural roadblocks such as the inability of young people to get business loans or the predilection of most youth for the stability and pensions that come with government jobs rather than the uncertainty and pressure of business careers. The number of built-in impediments to discourage young people from innovation was surprising.

Like it or not, though, change is upon us. Conservative countries may be further behind, but they are struggling with it, too. The staid nations of Western Europe face multiple financial, immigration, and security issues. China and Russia grapple with how far to move from highly centralized systems to free market states and democratic elections. China and India wrestle with explosive growth. Islamic nations try to balance traditional religious beliefs with a desire for democracy, a higher standard of living, and other benefits of modernity. The Middle East is being roiled by a younger generation tired of the old ways. As the saying goes, the only constant is change.

THE NEED FOR STABILITY ANCHORS

Extensive research into the effects of stress shows indisputably that the only good way for us to deal with it, especially if it's caused by change, is by having one or more areas in our lives that are completely stress free: stability zones. A stability zone (also known as stability anchor) is more than a physical location, though a place for quiet meditation is a bonus. It refers to some major feature of our lives that—in its constancy and dependability—helps ground us. An obvious example is the family, but that is what is most endangered in the modern world. Other immutable anchors are our moral principles and our commitment to our neighbors and community.

The importance of stability anchors is best demonstrated by what happens when they are missing. A perfect snapshot comes in the regular self-destruction of young movie stars and musicians. Assaulted by sudden change in the form of instant wealth and fame, they too often succumb to riotous living and chemical addictions. Those celebrities who survive and continue to grow as human beings invariably cite something that keeps them grounded: longtime friends; regular trips to their hometown, or even a residence there; hideaways where they can escape pressure. Pop icon Queen Latifah cites her native state as a major stability anchor for her: "There's something about growing up in New Jersey that prepares you for whatever you might encounter in the real world. We're not afraid to go places." She tells other people who are in the spotlight and therefore constantly stressed: "Make sure you have a sanctuary, because everybody in the world is going to be in your business." Even our accent can be an anchor for stability. Being from New Jersey, Arkansas, or Israel creates an immediate identity for anyone we meet.

A sense of ethnic or national identity can be our anchor in unfamiliar places, provided that it is not so strong that it leads to xenophobia. It is a small but terrible step to go from "my side is great" to "yours is terrible." All of us should carry enough of our native culture to bolster our identity but not enough to make us unwilling to accept the validity of, or to explore, other cultures. Americans have a strong belief in the U.S. Constitution. The British have a strong sense of tradition and cultural continuity, though China with its 4,000-year-old history likely has the longest tradition on which to base its modern identity. The French and Italians pride themselves on their countries' art and culture. These perspectives shape our thoughts and provide a strong base from which we can step forth into the world.

The beliefs of the people we respect can also shape our behavior and personal sense of identity. A young man who grew up without a father admired an early employer and chose to emulate this individual as he made his way up in the world. Role models and mentors, we call these. Even a negative stability anchor can provide a useful frame of reference. One young man left the South during a time of racial turmoil. Many people assumed by his accent that he was racist. He sought to prove them wrong. Years later, some of his friends referred to him in a positive way as a Southern gentleman. He sought to prove them right. A woman was torn by her relationship with her mother, who gave approval grudgingly but who also taught the woman many good traits, such as a strong work ethic and lovely social graces. The woman could not reconcile the contradictory aspects of her mother's personality and how they hurt her, until a friend told her: "Use the good stuff. Throw away the bad." This simple advice was liberating. She chose the anchors that helped her and released the ones that held her back. In the future, she tried less to please her mother, and was happier for it.

Along with our cultural heritage, each of us has a cache of stories about ourselves that we think about—and tell to others. These oft-repeated stories become a large measure of who we are. Because every one of our stories is unique to us, they give us a sense of self and stability. Our central image of ourselves might be that of a rags-to-riches workaholic, wonderful parent, top employee, philanthropist, protector of the environment, Walter Mitty sports hero, thoughtful lover, or devoted spouse. How much these stories mean to us becomes painfully clear when that image shatters; when, for example, the devoted wife learns that her husband wants a divorce, or when the husband and breadwinner of thirty years loses his job to the great recession.

For this reason, our self-image should be rooted in who we are intrinsically rather than in our relationships to others. The stories must also be positive. Anchors should stabilize us, not drag us down. Mental health professionals are constantly working to help troubled individuals rebuild their self-image by changing the stories they tell about themselves. We may also need to update these stories from time to time. The jilted wife, for instance, might begin a new story about the strong and independent woman who can make it on her own. The laid-off husband might begin a new story of the entrepreneur who starts a new business at age fifty.

The uncommitted can survive and prosper by discarding jobs, geography, and relationships. But they cannot discard everything. Cherished stories, however minor, carry a lot of weight. They are part and parcel of our identity. Providing a sense of coherence, they go with us everywhere we go.

Providing ourselves with positive stories does not simply make us feel better or more secure. When they are new, these stories recast our mental connections. They literally rewire the brain. These changes do not banish our troubles, but they do give us the mental energy and psychic resilience to tackle life's challenges.

If we have a core belief system, and a core set of people and relationships we believe in and are emotionally anchored to, then we have more freedom to change other aspects of our lives. Much as a child needs a strong parental bond in order to feel safe enough to explore the surrounding world, an adult needs to feel safe in core psychological areas in order to cope with the stress of experimentation. In our ever-changing, new-fashioned way of living, these old-fashioned concepts will help the center hold and keep anarchy from being loosed upon the world.

If much of this chapter has focused on sociological issues, society is driven by individual behavior, and individual behavior is driven by cognitive states. The point is that too much individual change can alter our cognitive processes in ways that collectively can have meaningful impact on society at large. As for the issue of uncommitted leaders, we must for now rely on observation and a bit of conjecture. It could be another example of life moving too fast for us as a species, or it might not prove to be a problem at all. Regardless, posing the question might help encourage the next generation to invest in traditional stability zones or to develop new kinds that work for them. If we want our leadership positions to be manned by human beings who are not total opportunists, we must encourage them to adopt anchors of stability against the winds of change.

══ LESSONS IN BRAINPOWER ══

- Given the tremendous effort required by most modern professions, people without commitments to family and community have a significant advantage over colleagues who have developed strong emotional roots.
- The uncommitted treat relationships, both personal and business, as being temporary and disposable. But leaders without ties are the ones most likely to make decisions that benefit themselves while hurting their organizations and communities.
- The way to avoid the stress of change and the rootlessness of the uncommitted is to develop stability anchors—things in our lives that give us a healthy psychological perspective from which to confront a confusing world.

EIGHTEEN

Leave Room Enough to Think

What would the world be like if we were all cognitively fit? At the minimum, the vast majority of us would live healthier and more interesting and productive lives. Increased brainpower would help us grapple with the complex questions and demands of our personal and public affairs . . . *with life itself*.

To achieve this brave new world, we will need to nourish an important skill: the ability to *unlearn* experience. And we will need to recapture the wonder and playfulness of a child . . . to reacquaint ourselves with the question "why?" The world runs on assumptions, which bury us in the past. Each new idea is born when someone ignores or challenges an assumption, yet this rarely happens until a calamity—usually crashing down from the outside—forces us to take a second look. When confronted by a problem, Toyota's founder developed the approach of asking "why" at least five times to ensure that he got past his assumptions and down to the root cause. Asking "why" from the seven different mental perspectives discussed in Chapter 14 can also lead us to new understanding of the real cause of a problem or of a possible solution.

A world of the cognitively fit would also be one in which all of us dive into and (largely) grasp important topics that are outside of our comfort zone. I once had the opportunity, along with a dozen other people, to spend a day with a group of astrophysicists. They gave an overview of their work and talked about many of the thorniest topics in their field: expanding or shrinking universe, black holes, dark matter, dark energy, quantum fluctuations, and so on. It was exciting to participate in a discussion that was so inherently interesting and yet so completely outside of my everyday concerns. Like my time in the immunology library, this experience invigorated my own mental energy for weeks to come.

Few of us are able to explore all of the wonderful subjects out there about which we have no clue. Even if we could expend the mental effort, the time required would make such an effort prohibitive. A cognitively fit world might provide job opportunities for people who could translate complex subjects for the general public. It is hard to imagine a more important role in a modern democracy than that of fairly and accurately presenting complex information in clear ways to the populace. Today, news broadcasts are home to empty sound bites—biased approaches to politics and stories about skateboarding squirrels. Newspaper-length articles are too short and too much of a snapshot to provide the necessary depth, and magazine articles too often take a single angle or hook in order to generate excitement and furor rather than to serve as a dispassionate reflection on the major issues. Books often provide a thoughtful perspective, but books are too time-intensive and detailed for consultation on every matter of interest. "Experts" often contradict one another. There's too much data, too much conflict, too much complexity, and too much specialized knowledge. The average citizen or legislator simply cannot make sense of it all. We need someone to explain all of the different angles in dispassionate, easy-to-comprehend language. An expert we know and trust!

Energy policy, for instance, is as confusing as it is critical to the future. What forms of energy are the safest or most dangerous, short term and long term? Are price differences the result of subsidies for the cheapest form, inefficiencies for the most expensive form—or a difference in volume that is affected by market incentives? Is it reasonable to develop new internal carbon sources in order to achieve energy independence? Are some carbon sources such as biomass acceptable because they reduce oil use as well as carbon pollution from forest fires?

Undoubtedly, a footnote-filled white paper lives somewhere in a dusty file or on the Internet that may answer these and other questions. Most of the information, however, is scattered and contradictory—much like the United States's energy policy itself. A contemporary search on "U.S. energy policy" returned *121 million results;* the first hundred or so results contained nothing that might answer these significant questions. That the largest energy-consuming nation has no national energy policy may well stem from the fact that no trusted, nontechnical voice has laid out all the options, considerations, and trade-offs in a way that regular citizens can understand and rally around.

Consider an Internet in which contributors provide thoughtful analysis on big topics instead of instant blogs on today's immediate news. Consider a Web in which the analysis almost always comes from someone we know, or at least someone we have come to trust, instead of an anonymous policy wonk from an unknown or partisan think tank. This quality of knowledge sharing is available on forums specific to certain fields or topics; the question is whether "social media 2.0" will bring it to the Web at large, on issues that matter to average citizens. We might ourselves become an "interpreter of truth" to our friends, explaining to them in detail a topic we personally care about.

A cognitively fit reader would not, of course, simply accept the findings of such an "arbiter" of truth. The reader would check at least some of the original research and would analyze the arguments and conclusions. Not everyone would agree with the findings, but the reasons for disagreement would be much clearer and based more on facts and less on posturing. A community of the cognitively fit would turn into a world in which every citizen contributes to the knowledge of others. A positive cycle of "gene times environment" would continue to raise the collective IQ. Everyone would retain rational skepticism about different viewpoints but would be willing to change position when new facts warrant it. If such a shift in mind-set seems utopian, the question is not whether it would happen but rather what would happen if it did.

Beyond any cognitive or psychological considerations, some kind of sea change is needed in how society addresses social and economic matters, business and politics, and local and global relations. The reason is that all of the easy questions—if there ever were any—have long since been answered. When only hard problems remain, only hard thinking will do.

KEEP AN OPEN MIND

One concept underlies the many lessons of this book. That is simply: Keep an open mind. Easy to say, hard to do. The good news is that the first step in avoiding automaticity is simply being aware of our tendency to slip into it. Knowing that we are prone to applying old formulas to new situations is often enough to release the mind, opening it to new possibilities. Intentionally identifying at least one new fact or consideration in a familiar-looking situation can change the context enough for us to see it with fresh eyes. Delaying important decisions gives the brain enough time to sort through all of the possibilities (both consciously and unconsciously).

Most people think they need to make critical decisions quickly. In reality this is seldom true. A thoughtful pause is often the best course of action. Aviators and doctors are trained not to react too fast in emergencies, because their instinctive choices may make the situation worse. Level the wings and keep the airspeed up, pilots learn, but otherwise avoid taking action until they really understand what's going on. In Abraham Vergese's lovely novel *Cutting for Stone,* an obstetrician involved in a terrifying emergency repeats to himself a surgeon's rule: "Think aloud . . . because it might help clarify the issues. . . . It was often the second mistake that came in haste to correct the first mistake that did the patient in." The same approach is valuable for many other complex decisions. Sometimes a scenario needs to sort itself out a bit before anyone can make sense of it. This is not to justify analysis paralysis but to avoid a panic-induced reaction, which usually makes a bad situation worse.

As we've seen, creativity stems from mental spontaneity. Throughout my career as a teacher, I never once gave a formal, prepared lecture. I would create a course syllabus and develop notes ahead of time on the topics I wanted to address in each class. The night before, I would review the points I wanted to make. When I stood before my students, I spoke extemporaneously. Even if a particular talk was not completely organized, the students were more captivated. They knew I was telling them *what I was thinking at that moment.* I was not regurgitating a talk I had given fifty times before. After a couple of years of teaching, when I knew the material really well, I would totally improvise. Sometimes this approach led to a completely different lecture. These talks were almost always the best. Thinking on my feet engaged me so much more than if I were reading from notes or repeating memorized text. Fresh ideas always emerged. My brain worked harder, and so did the brains of my students. This approach has caused me problems at conferences, however. After giving a speech, I am thanked by the organizer and asked for a written copy to put in the conference proceedings. "What written copy?" I say.

Since the age of thirty I have also taken no photographs—even on journeys to my beloved Africa. Photographs have been called memories frozen in time. That is just the problem: They freeze the memory into what the photo shows and nothing more. If we take a photo, the trip is over. The photo reminds us of the place, but it is not the memory of the place. We want the memory to stay alive, to keep working, to make more connections. Some people might claim that photos trigger memories rather than restrict them, though I tend to disagree. The discussion itself is thought provoking. And maybe the occasional documentary photo is appropriate, for example when family members come together or children reach life milestones. (A confession: Though I do not take such photos myself, I have on rare occasions asked others to! Sometimes a photo is enough.)

A similar freezing effect occurs with the stories we tell. We (automatically!) begin to create a beginning, a middle, and an end. The second time we tell a story, we recall it the way we told it before, not the way it necessarily happened. The more recent memory of the organized story supersedes the original. *Once we tell a story, we no longer remember the memory.* The original is lost. Like a photo, the memory becomes frozen, only this time in words.

Of course, people love to tell stories. As discussed in the previous chapter, these stories can become an important part of our identity. I'm not suggesting that we should stop telling stories, I'm suggesting that we postpone converting memories into stories for as long as possible. Recall the restricting effect of consciousness. Let memory, which is hidden, diffuse, and rich in imagery and sensation, process the information for as long as possible. Let the unconscious connect it with other memories in wonderful, unpredictable ways. The moment we structure an experience, it becomes an overlay to the original memory. We lose the raw material. This book is a story, of course. I put it off for many years to let its contents simmer.

All of us can find ways to free our thinking. This could make a good homework assignment. With every important project and decision, find at least one way to go off on a new track, *especially* if it deviates from the previous plan. When my daughter began to teach, she asked for advice. I said, "Don't overprepare. Leave yourself room enough to think."

FINAL THOUGHTS

We all live double lives. First, there is our external reality, the outside world and all the harm or happiness it may bring. Unforgiving or easy, this reality often operates outside of our control. Then, there is also our own separate, personal life of the mind. In this interior life, we react to immediate events and develop long-term coping strategies. We create, combine, and recombine new thoughts and ideas. We feel love and heartbreak, sympathy and anger—every emotion that makes us human. We not only respond to external stimuli, but we also create our own reality. Our private interior lives exist in the near-instantaneous calculations and thoughts of our brain, working upon a body of knowledge and emotional memories that's built over a lifetime. We build the profundity of consciousness out of nothing—or at least, out of nothing more glorious than exceedingly complex chemistry.

Cogito ergo sum: René Descartes' famous line, "I think, therefore I am." The "I" in that statement is the internal voice we constantly hear in our heads. Our mental existence is defined by this nonstop interior monologue. Our closest companion is not our loving spouse, parent, child, or friend, but our own mind—our best and most constant companion. If that internal narrative breaks down, then the "I" does not exist anymore. Thinking must be organized. If we cannot cohere our thoughts and ideas, then "I" am dust in the wind.

Thoughts must also have context. Without a past or future, thoughts have no meaning. They are just babble. Memories create personal histories that form the basis for our interactions with other people and also for culture and civilization. Memories enable us to take our place among the thousands of generations of people who came before and (we surely hope) will follow. If we lose our memories, we can neither learn nor treasure our history over time. We have no way to gauge the pros and cons of actions. We have no way to maintain personal bonds and associations. We are not merely babbling, we are lost at sea. If thinking is what creates our special existence, then memories provide the *meaning* of our lives.

That is the tragedy of Alzheimer's and other degenerative diseases of the brain. We first lose our memories and then our ability to function in the here and now. We lose ourselves . . . our *selves*. We are alone in a way that no human being should ever be. This is why we all have deep-rooted anxieties about the health of our brain. This is why building and maintaining our cognitive health is so critical.

Cognitive fitness involves preparing our minds for the contest of life and bringing our best mental energies to bear on the most difficult personal and professional issues that confront us in life. The goal is to develop better ways of handling the multiple and often conflicting circumstances that are a part of life. By understanding the brain and its ability to change functionally and biologically, we should be able to avoid the pitfalls of our inherently conservative nature and take advantage of the great creativity that lies within. Built on the brain's plasticity, cognitive fitness must become a defining aspect of our lives. Because the brain creates both our physical and psychological reality, cognitive fitness radiates outward into the external world. Consequently, *Maximum Brainpower* has stretched from the innermost workings of the mind to the outermost impact

MENTAL JOG VERSUS MENTAL WORKOUT

We cannot be a "weekend warrior" with our brains any more than with our bodies. The difference between casual cognitive work and a brainpower regimen is this:

- Reading an occasional book versus taking a class in literature or actively participating in a book club.
- Listening to an occasional language tape versus taking a formal language course or speaking a new language at home several times a week.
- Plinking on a piano once in a while versus taking regular lessons or playing with a group.
- Texting, posting on a social network, or writing an occasional email, versus keeping a detailed and thoughtful diary.
- Casually pursuing a hobby versus making it an avocation. Amateurs have made major contributions to astronomy, atmospheric science, biology, ornithology, and other fields. Example: A Dutch schoolteacher found a green blob of galactic gas that is now the subject of formal astronomical study. Sewing, mechanics, woodworking: Any area of interest done conscientiously will benefit the brain.
- Occasional Internet browsing versus intense, thoughtful research. Further, the collaborative nature of the wired world has encouraged average citizens to participate in a variety of social, political, and other projects. Collaborative online reading may be a useful wrinkle for an otherwise solitary pursuit—as long as digital book clubs do not replace "live" book clubs.

they have on society. Many books take a single idea and hammer it throughout. We have interwoven many ideas involving many different contexts. All of those ideas, though, come back to the brain. If we understand the brain, we understand the world. If we can improve the brain, we can change the world.

Early on, my discussions about this project led to the question: Where on the spectrum of knowledge is our understanding of the brain? As a comparison, a colleague said he would put today's computer and Internet technologies at about where airplanes were in the 1930s. In other words, it will take several more intellectual leaps before digital technology reaches a comfortable maturity. Well, I said, if today's computers are the equivalent of a 1930s airplane, then today's brain science is the equivalent of an 1850 railroad. We are not so far from understanding the brain as one recent skeptic claimed, saying, "*All* problems in neuroscience are unsolved." We know a good deal about brain biology. New technologies have dramatically improved our understanding of the physical, chemical, and electrical activity within the brain. We understand how the brain works on the cellular level and much about how the parts of the nervous system work together. Scientists are beginning to correlate a large body of experiential observation of human behavior directly with the physical functioning of the brain itself. Though we are nowhere close to taking flight, we have laid down solid tracks toward the future. Come join in the journey. The real fun is still ahead.

Acknowledgments

Shlomo Breznitz:
I am greatly indebted to many, but I wish to thank my teacher, Pinchas Blumenthal, for opening my eyes, Sonny Kugelmass for leading me into research, and Michael Kaplan for making it possible.

Shlomo Breznitz and Collins Hemingway:
Thanks, first, to our agent, Glen Hartley of Writers' Representatives. He not only took on *Maximum Brainpower* but his initial thoughts on the book helped shape our overall approach and organization. To Beth Rashbaum, the editor who enthusiastically selected our book for Ballantine Bantam Dell. To Angela Polidoro, who diligently edited the manuscript through three successive passes. Angela's observations, both strategic and tactical, made the text much more approachable, and her suggestions and tough questions helped clarify many of the more difficult examples and passages. To our copyeditor, Angela Pica, for her sharp eye; to Crystal Velasquez, who led us through the production process; and the entire team at Ballantine Bantam Dell.

To Leo Goldberger, Wendy Hemingway, and Jody Peake for their feedback during manuscript development. To Linda O'Neill, especially, for offering detailed substantive commentary far beyond what we could have expected from a colleague or friend. To Chris Schweppe and Ben Benson of the Mandala Agency for their quick turnaround and quality work on graphic images. To Anthony Maulucci for his generous permission to let us quote his poetry.

A number of people helped shape and improve the work. Any weaknesses or errors in the text remain solely the responsibility of the authors.

Bibliography

Arum, Richard, and Josipa Roksa. *Academically Adrift: Limited Learning on College Campuses.* Chicago: University of Chicago Press, 2011.

Begley, Sharon. *Train Your Mind, Change Your Brain: How a New Science Reveals Our Extraordinary Potential to Transform Ourselves.* New York: Ballantine Books, 2007.

Breznitz, Shlomo. *Cry Wolf: The Psychology of False Alarms.* Hillsdale, N. J.: Lawrence Erlbaum Associates, 1984.

Breznitz, Shlomo. *Denial of Stress.* New York: International Universities Press, 1983.

Breznitz, Shlomo. The effect of hope on coping with stress. In M. Appley & R. Trumbull (Eds.), *Dynamics of Stress.* New York: Plenum, 1986.

Dickens, W. T., and J. R. Flynn. "Heritability Estimates Versus Large Environmental Effects: The IQ Paradox Resolved." *Psychological Review* 108, no. 2 (2001): 346–69.

Doidge, Norman. *The Brain That Changes Itself: Stories of Personal Triumph from the Frontiers of Brain Science.* New York: Viking Penguin, 2007.

Dreyfus, Hubert L., and Stuart Dreyfus. "From Socrates to Expert Systems: The Limits of Calculative Rationality." In *Interpretive Social Science, a Second Look,* by eds. Paul Rabinow and William Sullivan. Berkeley: University of California Press, 1987.

Edelman, Gerald M. *Neural Darwinism: The Theory of Neuronal Group Selection*. New York: Basic Books, 1987.

Fox, Douglas. "The Limits of Intelligence." *Scientific American,* July 2011: 37–43.

Freud, Sigmund, translated and edited by A. A. Brill. *The Basic Writings of Sigmund Freud (Psychopathology of Everyday Life, the Interpretation of Dreams, and Three Contributions to the Theory of Sex)*. New York: Modern Library Edition, Random House, 1995.

"Functional Fixedness." Wikipedia. July 1, 2010. http://en.wikipedia.org/wiki/Functional_fixedness (accessed August 5, 2010).

Gardner, Howard. *Multiple Intelligences: New Horizons in Theory and Practice*. New York: Basic Books, 2006.

Gawande, Atul. *The Checklist Manifesto: How to Get Things Right*. New York: Metropolitan Books, 2009.

Gay, Peter. *Freud: A Life for Our Time*. New York: W. W. Norton, 1988.

Gazzaniga, Michael S., Richard B. Ivry, and George R. Mangun. *Cognitive Neuroscience: The Biology of the Mind*. New York: W. W. Norton & Company, 2008.

German, Tim P., and Margaret Anne Defeyter. "Immunity to Functional Fixedness in Young Children." *Psychonomic Bulletin & Review,* 2000: 707–12.

Gigerenzer, Gerd. *Gut Feelings: The Intelligence of the Unconscious*. New York: Penguin Books, 2007.

Gladwell, Malcolm. *Blink*. New York: Little, Brown and Company, 2005.

Goldberg, Elkhonon. *The Wisdom Paradox*. London: Pocket Books, 2007.

Goldberger, Leo, and Shlomo Breznitz. *Handbook of Stress: Theoretical and Clinical Aspects,* 2nd edition. New York: The Free Press, 1993.

Gorlick, Adam. "Media Multitaskers Pay Mental Price, Stanford Study Shows." *Stanford Report,* August 2009.

Greenwood, P. M., and R. Parasuraman. "Neuronal and Cognitive Plasticity: A Neurocognitive Framework for Ameliorating Cognitive Aging." *Front. Ag. Neurosci.,* no. 2 (2010): 150.

Heckscher, Charles, Saul Rubinstein, Linda Flynn, Niclas Erhardt, and Boniface Michael. "Collaboration and the Quality of Health Care Delivery." http://mitsloan.mit.edu/iwer/pdf/0809-heckscher.pdf. Draft: April 17, 2008.

Holland, Earle. "Stress of Breast Cancer Surgery, Diagnosis Weakens Immune System." *The Ohio State University Research*. January 7, 1998. http://researchnews.osu.edu/archive/barb.htm (accessed June 18, 2010).

"Holmes and Rahe Stress Scale." Wikipedia. February 1, 2011. http://en .wikipedia.org/wiki/Holmes_and_Rahe_stress_scale (accessed June 28, 2011).

Horowitz-Kraus, Tzipi, and Zvia Breznitz. "Can the Error Detection Mechanism Benefit from Training the Working Memory? A Comparison between Dyslexics and Controls." *PLoS ONE* 4 (9): www.plosone .org/article/infoidoi%2F10.1371%2Fjournal.pone.0007141 September 2009.

James, William. *Writings 1902–1910: The Varieties of Religious Experience / Pragmatism / A Pluralistic Universe / The Meaning of Truth / Some Problems of Philosophy / Essays (Library of America)*. New York: Penguin Books, 1987.

Jung, Carl. *The Undiscovered Self*. New York: SIGNET, 2006.

Kramer, Arthur F., Kirk K. Erickson, and Stanley J. Colcombe. "Exercise, Cognition, and the Aging Brain." *Journal of Applied Physiology*, 2006: 1,237–42.

Kroger, Edeltraut, Ross Andel, Joan Lindsay, Zohra Benounissa, Rene Verreault, and Danielle Laurin. "Is Complexity of Work Associated with Risk of Dementia? The Canadian Study of Health and Aging." *Am J Epidemiol* 167, no. 7 (2008): 820–30.

Langa, Kenneth M., et al. "Cognitive Health Among Older Adults in the United States and in England." *BioMed Central*. June 25, 2009. http:// www.biomedcentral.com/1471–2318/9/23 (accessed August 23, 2010).

Lazarus, Richard. *Psychological Stress and the Coping Process*. New York: McGraw-Hill, 1966.

Luchins, Abraham S., with Edith H. Luchins. *Rigidity of Behavior: A Variational Approach to the Effect of Einstellung*. Eugene, OR: University of Oregon Press, 1959.

Maguire, Eleanor A., David G. Gadian, Ingrid S. Johnsrude, Catriona D. Good, John Ashburner, Richard S. J. Frackowiak, and Christopher D. Fri. "Navigation-Related Structural Change in the Hippocampi of Taxi Drivers." *PNAS* 97, no. 8 (April 2000): 4,398–4,403.

Maulucci, A. S. *100 Love Sonnets*. Lorenzo Press, 2007. www.lorenzo-press.com. See also http://www.anthonymaulucci.com/home-writing .html.

Merzenich, Michael, and Josef Syka. "Plasticity and Signal Representation in the Auditory System." *Proceedings of the International Symposium on Plasticity of the Central Auditory System and the Processing of Complex Acoustic Signals.* Prague, Czech Republic: Springer, 2003.

Minsky, Marvin. *The Society of Mind.* New York: Simon & Schuster, 1987.

Nisbett, Richard, and Timothy Wilson. "Telling More Than We Can Know: Verbal Reports on Mental Processes." *Psychological Review* 84, no. 3 (May 1977): 231–57.

Nithianantharajah, J., and A. J. Hannan. "The Neurobiology of Brain and Cognitive Reserve: Mental and Physical Activity as Modulators of Brain Disorders." *Prog Neurobiol,* December 2009: 369–82.

Owen, Adrian. "Does Brain Training Really Work?" September 7, 2009. http://news.bbc.co.uk/2/hi/uk_news/8237945.stm (accessed September 13, 2009).

Peterson, Christopher, Stephen F. Maier, and Martin E. P. Seligman. *Learned Helplessness: A Theory for the Age of Personal Control.* New York: Oxford University Press, 1995.

Pfeiffer, John E. *The Emergence of Man.* New York: Harper & Row, 1978.

Phillips, David P., et al. "Cardiac Mortality Spikes on Christmas and New Year's." *Circulation.* http://circ.ahajournals.org/cgi/content/full/110/25/3781, no. 110 (2004): 3,781–88.

Phillips, David P., and Daniel G. Smith. "Postponement of Death Until Symbolically Meaningful Occasions." *JAMA* 263, no. 14 (April 1990).

Piaget, Jean. *The Psychology of the Child.* New York: Basic Books, 1972.

Rogers, Heather, and Juan Carlos Arango Lasprilla. "Retrogenesis Theory in Alzheimer's Disease: Evidence and Clinical Implications." *Anales de Psicologia,* December 2006: 260–66.

Schaie, K. W. *Developmental Influences on Adult Intelligence: The Seattle Longitudinal Study.* New York: Oxford University Press, 2005.

Segerstrom, Suzanne, and Gregory E. Miller. "Psychological Stress and the Human Immune System: A Meta-Analytic Study of 30 Years of Inquiry." *Psychological Bulletin,* 2004: 601–30.

Seligman, Martin E. P. *Learned Optimism.* New York: Knopf, 1990.

Selye, Hans. *Stress Without Distress.* New York: SIGNET, 1978.

Shimizu, Mitsuri, and Bret Pelham. "Postponing a Date with the Grim Reaper: Ceremonial Events, the Will to Live, and Mortality." *Basic and Applied Social Psychology* 30 (2008): 36–45.

Singer, P. W. *Wired for War: The Robotics Revolution and Conflict in the 21st Century.* New York: The Penguin Press, 2009.

Snowdon, David. *Aging With Grace: What the Nun Studies Teach Us About Living Longer, Healthier, and More Meaningful Lives.* New York: Bantam, 2001.

Spence, Donald. "Conscious and Preconscious Influences on Recall: Another Example of the Restricting Effects of Awareness." *The Journal of Abnormal and Social Psychology* 68, no. 1 (January 1964): 92–99.

Stern, Yaakov. "Cognitive Reserve and Alzheimer's Disease." *Alzheimer Dis Assoc Disord* 20, no. 2 (April–June 2006).

Stouffer, Samuel Andrew. *The American Soldier: Studies in Social Psychology in World War II.* Princeton: Princeton University Press, 1949.

Taylor, Jill Bolte. *My Stroke of Insight: A Brain Scientist's Personal Journey.* New York: Viking Penguin, 2008.

Turkheimer, Eric. "Socioeconomic Status Modifies Heritability of IQ in Young Children." *Psychol Sci* 14 (November 2003): 623–28.

Urcuioli, Peter J. "Categorization & Acquired Equivalence." n.d. http://www.pigeon.psy.tufts.edu/avc/urcuioli/default.htm (accessed November 18, 2010).

Von Domarus, E. "The Specific Laws of Logic in Schizophrenia." In *Language and Thought in Schizophrenia*, by J. S. Kasanin (ed.), 104–13. Berkeley: University of California Press, 1944.

Wade, Nicholas. "Decoding the Human Brain." *The New York Times,* December 13, 2010.

Whalley, Lawrence, et al. "Cognitive Reserve and the Neurobiology of Cognitive Aging." *Ageing Research Reviews,* 2004: 369–82.

General Topics of Interest

Since one of our purposes is to encourage in-depth exploration and independent thought, we wish to point readers to the many general topics of interest covered in the book. A world of material exists online that can be found by searching almost any keyword related to the main concepts discussed, but particularly the following keywords:

Alzheimer's disease, dementia
Anniversary effect
Artificial intelligence, AI
Brain, adult neurogenesis
Brain development
Brain health
Brain, multitasking
Brain plasticity
Brain scans or PET scans
Cognitive fitness
Cognitive reserve
Exercise and the brain

Improvised explosive devices, IED
Insect brain
Intelligence quotient, IQ
Neuroscience
Pigeon intelligence
Placebo effect
Schizophrenia
Stress
Videogames and the brain
Word association
Work-life balance, working hours
Yom Kippur War

Index

ABOUT THE AUTHORS

PROFESSOR SHLOMO BREZNITZ is an internationally renowned psychologist who has more than thirty years of research experience in the field of stress and cognition. He has served as a visiting professor at the University of California at Berkeley, Stanford University, London School of Economics, Rockefeller University, the National Institutes of Health of the U.S. Department of Health and Human Services, and other leading institutions. He is founding director of the Center for the Study of Psychological Stress at the University of Haifa, where he has also served as Lady Davis Professor of Psychology, Rector, and University President.

Author of six academic books and many scientific articles, Professor Breznitz has also written *Memory Fields,* a well-regarded memoir of his family's experiences during the Holocaust, and recently completed his autobiography.

At an age when most people retire, Professor Breznitz founded CogniFit, a company that has won several awards for software products that improve cognitive fitness. In addition to his academic and business career, Professor Breznitz has also served in the Israeli Parliament.

COLLINS HEMINGWAY is a writer and technologist whose range of interests is shown in the books on which he has collaborated. He is co-author with Microsoft CEO Bill Gates of the #1 bestselling book on business and technology, *Business @ the Speed of Thought;* co-author with Dan Baker and Cathy Greenberg on *What Happy Companies Know,* about how positive cultures help companies outperform competitors; co-author with Arthur Rubinfeld on *Built for Growth,* the gold standard about how companies can create and renew retail brands; and consultant on books ranging from supply-chain management to leadership and business strategies. He has also written on a variety of other topics, including aviation, medicine, and emerging technologies.

ABOUT THE TYPE

This book was set in Sabon, a typeface designed by the well-known German typographer Jan Tschichold (1902–74). Sabon's design is based upon the original letter forms of Claude Garamond and was created specifically to be used for three sources: foundry type for hand composition, Linotype, and Monotype. Tschichold named his typeface for the famous Frankfurt typefounder Jacques Sabon, who died in 1580.